PHYSICAL EXAMINATION IN ORTHOPAEDICS

PHYSICAL EXAMINATION IN ORTHOPAEDICS

A. Graham Apley
MB BS FRCS FRCSEd(Hon)

Consulting Orthopaedic Surgeon,
St Thomas's Hospital, London.
Emeritus Consultant Surgeon,
Rowley Bristow Orthopaedic Hospital, Pyrford,
and St Peter's Hospital Chertsey, Surrey.
Former Editor, British Issue,
Journal of Bone and Joint Surgery

Louis Solomon
MBChB MD FRCS FRCSEd

Emeritus Professor of Orthopaedic Surgery,
University of Bristol.
Formerly Professor of Orthopaedic Surgery,
University of the Witwatersrand,
Johannesburg

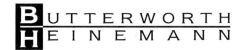

Butterworth- Heinemann
Linacre House, Jordan Hill, Oxford OX2 8DP
A division of Reed Educational and Professional Publishing Ltd

℞ A member of the Reed Elsevier plc group

OXFORD BOSTON JOHANNESBURG
MELBOURNE NEW DELHI SINGAPORE

First published 1997
© Reed Educational and Professional Publishing Ltd 1997

British Library Cataloguing in the Publication Data

A catalogue record for this book is available from the British Library

ISBN 0 7506 1766 7

Printed and bound in Scotland by Cambus Litho Ltd, Glasgow

CONTENTS

ACKNOWLEDGEMENTS

We are deeply grateful to our two models, Sheila Breeze and Keith James, who endured the discomfort and tedium of posing for most of the illustrations. Their experience as senior physiotherapists ensured that they understood exactly what we were trying to show in each picture, and this made our task immeasurably easier.

Equally patient was our photographer, Elizabeth Hurst, who remained unruffled by our frequent demands to 'try another angle' or 'shoot from above'; occasionally she had to repeat the entire 'shoot'. To her, our thanks.

We also hasten to acknowledge our indebtedness to the patients who allowed us to photograph them and use the pictures in our teaching and training courses. In addition to coping with the discomforts and anxieties of their illness, they willingly put up with the cold gaze of cameras. Theirs is an invaluable contribution to medical education.

Finally, we owe more than we can ever repay to those students and trainees who, over the years, have stimulated us to go on producing books such as this one. They have been the source of deep fulfilment in our work as teachers and trainers.

A. G. A.
L. S.

Preface

Generations of doctors have warned that the art of clinical examination is dying – and they have always been right; the problem is progressive disuse atrophy. Imaging and other investigations have so much to contribute to diagnosis that the whole of it is often put upon their shoulders. Moreover, the medical school curriculum has become so overloaded that practical skills such as history taking and clinical examination are being crowded out. That is the *raison d'être* of this book.

It is often supposed that clinical examination begins on the couch. Not so – it begins as the patient enters the room. You can see at a glance whether the person is tall or short, fat or thin, ill or well, energetic or slow. As he or she approaches, you notice the gait and any obvious deformities. After the usual greeting, you should see that your patient is seated comfortably before your dialogue and examination begin.

The art of clinical examination has to be learnt – it does not come naturally. This seems obvious, but though you may be shown how to use your hands for operating, have you been shown how to use them for examining? Or, for that matter, how to position yourself and the patient? We have addressed this question by arranging our material as a sequential series of pictures and captions showing one good way of handling each stage of the examination.

The system we advocate, and which we ourselves practise, is based upon three imperatives: *look*, *feel* and *move*.

Looking comes first, and of course continues while we feel and while we are examining movements. It requires stern self-discipline to refrain from touching a lump the moment you see it, but once you put your hand on it you switch off visual information.

Feeling is not a process of casual stroking or pointless prodding. It should be methodical, encompassing first the skin, then the peri-articular structures, then the joint capsule, the synovium and its contents (especially testing for the presence of fluid) and then the bones.

When we feel a lump we note its boundaries, the character of its edge, its surface, consistency and local attachments. Feeling for tenderness needs special care, so that we may detect the slight change of expression when we are beginning to cause pain. Right-handed examiners see the patient's face better if they stand on the patient's right; if you are left-handed you should stand on the left.

Movement can be active, passive or abnormal. The advantage of beginning with active movements is that you can see at what point the patient begins to feel pain; then, when you examine passive movements you know when to be particularly careful. When possible show the patient what to do, and at all times use words which will be understood – 'bend' rather than 'flex', 'straighten' rather than 'extend', and so on.

By the time the clinical examination is complete, you should have a fair idea of the diagnosis – or at least the differential diagnosis. Only then can you enter intelligently on the next stage of the diagnostic journey: imaging, laboratory investigations or special tests aimed at confirming or excluding a specific abnormality. Remember, though, that clinical examination is not *only* about diagnosis. It is the introduction to a unique relationship. It may sometimes feel like an exercise in detection, but heaven forbid that you should behave like a sleuth and forget your role as a doctor. Talking and listening, feeling the affected part, keeping eye contact, handling the painful limb without hurting the patient – all this has as much to do with *care* as with diagnosis.

THE CLINICAL ENCOUNTER

Diagnosis, according to the dictionary, is the identification of disease from symptoms and signs. In a caring society, it has come to mean much more: it is the recognition and understanding not only of a specific *abnormality* but also of the *loss of function* and the general *disability* arising from it. Making 'spot diagnoses' may be fun, but full understanding evolves only from a concerned dialogue with the patient and careful, systematic examination and investigation.

THE SETTING

You may see your patient for the first time in a consulting room, an outpatient clinic, their own home, a ward bed or a trolley in the casualty department. The physical setting may vary, but what really matters is the ambience which you create in that encounter.

Patients should feel at ease and assured of respect and confidentiality; if the clinic is 'open', it should be arranged so that adjacent groups cannot overhear each other. Patients need to have their complaints taken seriously, and the diagnosis or proposed treatment explained in terms which are neither patronizing nor overloaded with scientific detail. Generate a sense of confidence by showing that you know exactly what you are doing.

TAKING A HISTORY

Talking with patients serves a double purpose: it elicits information and it is also therapeutic. Patients need to tell, and they need to be heard. So let them speak and tell their story.

'Taking a history' is a misnomer. The patient tells a story; it is we the listeners who construct a history, from entrenched narratives, anecdotes, parables and family myths.

··

The story may be maddeningly disorganized; the history has to be systematic. We have followed a particular scheme in this book, listing the complaints that come up most frequently: pain, stiffness, swelling, deformity, instability, weakness, altered sensation and loss of function. Remember, though, that each of these symptoms needs to be picked over for further information. When did it start? Did something, possibly an injury, trigger it? Did it come on suddenly or gradually? What makes it worse, or better? Are others in the family affected?

Then there is the matter of interpretation. What do these symptoms, or complaints, really mean?

Pain

This is the most common symptom in orthopaedics. Listen to the patient's description and try to establish exactly where it is, when it comes on, how often it is felt and how severe it is; you will learn a great deal, not only about the nature of the disorder but also about the patient's life and feelings of care or neglect. Above all, remember two things: (a) patients have not learnt anatomy; when they say 'The pain is in my shoulder' it could be in the shoulder joint, the acromio-clavicular joint, the rotator cuff, the humerus or the deltoid muscle. Ask them to point, if possible, to the exact site of greatest intensity. And (b) pain from deep structures is poorly localized and usually 'referred' elsewhere; thus, pain in the vicinity of the shoulder may be referred from the neck, and true shoulder joint pain may appear lower down in the arm.

Stiffness

Patients often find it difficult to distinguish stiffness from lack of movement due to pain; be sure that you and your patient are speaking about the same thing. Also enquire whether 'stiff' means totally or partially restricted.

Swelling

Swelling may be in the soft tissues, the joint or the bone; to the patient they are all the same. Record the information but reserve judgement on what is swollen until you examine the part. Don't dismiss the complaint; patients are seldom wrong about something being swollen. Even if the area doesn't *look* swollen, it probably is, and the patient senses it because the skin feels tight or perhaps a ring or a shoe doesn't fit as loosely as before.

Deformity

'Vanity, thy name is woman' (and man and child!). Many deformities (round shoulders, knock knees, bandy legs, flat feet, pigeon toes, knobbly fingers) may not seem very serious, but to the patient and his family they are important. Learn to recognize which ones really matter: a crooked spine, a joint that won't straighten, a bone that was formerly straight and only recently became bent. Any *progressive* deformity obviously needs attention.

Weakness

Weakness is a very vague symptom. Try to pin the patient down to a precise description; if one specific movement (or set of movements) is weak and the others quite normal, this is a valuable clue, possibly to neurological disorder.

Instability

Patients don't use that term. They speak of a joint 'giving way'. This may be due to muscle weakness or dysfunction of the ligaments holding the joint. More dramatic complaints of a part 'coming out of joint' should be carefully assessed. A shoulder or a patella may indeed dislocate spontaneously; a hip, never.

Change in sensibility

Numbness or tingling suggests injury, localized pressure, entrapment or ischaemia anywhere along the course of the nerve. Try to establish its exact distribution, because this will tell you where the fault lies. If multiple sites are affected, this may signify a peripheral neuropathy. Symptoms that are described only vaguely ('my whole arm goes dead') should be interpreted only after physical examination.

Loss of function

Always ask the patient how their symptoms interfere with their activities. Loss of movement in the index finger means far less to a lawyer than to a concert violinist (or, for that matter, to a chicken plucker!). Athletes and sports people are the most demanding of all. What sounds like a fairly trivial problem to an unsympathetic doctor may spell the end of someone's career.

Past history and family history

Patients may either omit mentioning previous illnesses or accidents because they don't appreciate their connection with the present complaint, or they may use the opportunity to unburden themselves of all their former troubles, relevant or not. This is where you must lead the interview and ask specifically about previous injuries or illnesses that could bear directly on the diagnosis.

The same goes for the family history. If a young man presents for the first time with a painful, tensely swollen knee and no history of any injury, it is important to ask about bleeding disorders among his relatives; the patient may not know that this is important unless he is prompted.

EXAMINING THE PATIENT

Some disorders cause symptoms which are so characteristic that you can make the diagnosis without examining the patient. Carpal tunnel syndrome is one example. In some other conditions, one glance is enough; who could mistake the hand deformities of rheumatoid arthritis for anything else? Nevertheless, even in these cases a systematic approach is worthwhile; you will acquire the habit and the patient will feel that he or she has been properly attended to.

Make sure that the parts to be examined are suitably exposed. Don't leave it to the patient to divine your intentions; give him or her precise instructions: for example 'Please take off your top clothes and keep your underclothes on so that I can examine your back'.

If one limb is affected, both must be exposed so that they can be compared. First examine the good limb, then the bad; only by proceeding in a purposeful, disciplined way can we avoid missing important signs.

The system we use is simple but comprehensive:

- LOOK

- FEEL

- MOVE

Look

We look first at the *skin* (especially for scars and colour changes); then at the *shape* (is there swelling or wasting?); and then at the *position* (is there any deformity?).

When describing deformity, it may seem pedantic to replace 'bow legs' and 'knock knees' with 'genu varum' and 'genu valgum', but such formality is justified by the need for clarity and consistency. *Varus* means that the part distal to the joint is deviated towards the midline, *valgus* away from it.

The term *fixed deformity* is ambiguous. It seems to mean that the joint is deformed and immobile. Not so – it means that one particular movement cannot be completed. Thus, if a knee can flex fully but cannot extend fully it is said to have a *fixed flexion deformity*.

Feel

Feeling is exploring, not groping aimlessly. If you know your anatomy, you know where to find the various landmarks. By following the map in your mind's eye you can tell if anything is out of place or mis-shapen.

Feeling for tenderness is crucial. While doing so, look at the patient's face, not at your hands (Figures **1.1** and **1.2**). You know where they are, or you should. Try to localize any tenderness to a particular structure; knowing *where* it is will often tell you *what* it is.

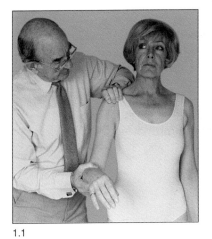

1.1

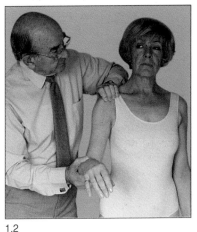

1.2

1.1 Feeling for tenderness – the wrong way

1.2 Feeling for tenderness – look at the patient's face, not your hands

Move

Ask the patient to move (*active movement*) before you move the joint (*passive movement*). This will give you an idea of the range of movement and whether it is painful or not.

By convention the range of movement is recorded in degrees, starting from zero, which is the neutral or anatomical position of the joint. For accuracy you can use a goniometer (Figure **1.3**), but with practice you will learn to estimate the angles by eye. What is important is to compare the symptomatic with the asymptomatic or normal side.

Describing the range of movement is often made to seem difficult. Words such as 'full', 'good', 'limited' and 'poor' are misleading. *Always cite the range or span, from start to finish, in degrees.* For example, 'Knee

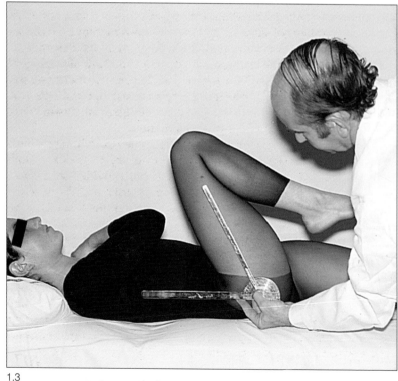

1.3

1.3 Using a goniometer to measure the range of hip flexion

flexion 0 – 140°' means that the range of flexion is from zero (the knee absolutely straight) through an arc of 140 degrees (the leg making an acute angle with the thigh). Similarly, 'Knee flexion 20 – 90°' means that the joint lacks the last 20 degrees of extension and it flexes only to a right angle.

Abnormal movement refers to movement which is inherently unphysiological. You may be able to shift or angulate a hinge joint, such as the knee, at right angles to the normal plane of movement; you may almost be able to reproduce a previous dislocation or subluxation; indeed, merely starting the movement which previously resulted in dislocation may be so distressing that the patient goes rigid with anxiety at the anticipated result – this is aptly called the *apprehension test*. These are all signs of instability.

Additional examination

The method followed here should be regarded as a guide, not a law engraved on tablets of stone. Sometimes we need to 'move' before we can properly 'look', for example when looking for spinal deformity.

In other cases the symptoms demand a full neurological assessment as the priority. Or we may wish to confirm or exclude one particular diagnosis by performing a special test (for example, the 'jerk test' or the 'pivot shift test' for cruciate ligament dysfunction) which has no application in any other situation.

The method will also need to be modified when examining patients with acute injuries. Obviously you would not try to 'move' a limb with a suspected fracture when an X-ray can provide the answer. Moreover, resuscitation will always take priority and in severely injured patients the detailed local examination may need to be curtailed or deferred.

Paediatric practice requires special skills. You may get no first-hand account of the symptoms; a baby screaming with pain will tell you very little, and over-anxious parents will probably tell you too much. When examining the child, you should be flexible. If he or she is moving a particular joint, take your opportunity to examine movement then and there. You will learn much more by adopting methods of play than by applying a rigid system of examination. And leave any test for tenderness until last!

Axioms

1. Make sure your patient is at ease and comfortable.
2. Give clear instructions as to what you want him or her to do.
3. Expose fully the area to be examined.
4. The limbs are symmetrical; always examine both and compare them.
5. Joints are three-dimensional; examine front, back and sides.
6. Look at your patient's face and not only at your hands.
7. Do not cause pain.
8. Repeating a test once or twice shows caution and wisdom; excessive repetition suggests that you are confused.
9. Talk to your patient and tell him or her what you have found.
10. Record everything, including a summary of what you have told your patient.

THE SHOULDER 2

HISTORY

Pain is the commonest symptom. But 'pain in the shoulder' is not necessarily 'shoulder pain'! If the patient points to the top of the shoulder, think of the acromioclavicular joint, or referred pain from the neck. Pain from the shoulder joint and the rotator cuff is felt, typically, over the front and outer aspect of the joint, often as far down as the insertion of the deltoid and occasionally even further.

Stiffness is important if it is persistent. It may become so severe as to merit the term *'frozen shoulder'* (not frozen cold, but frozen stiff); however, this term is more correctly reserved for a specific syndrome of prolonged pain and stiffness which is probably a type of reflex sympathetic dystrophy.

Deformity is seldom noticed until it is marked; for example, prominence of the scapula ('winging'), or a tendency to hold the arm in a fixed position.

Instability symptoms may be gross and alarming: the shoulder 'jumps out of its socket' when the patient abducts and externally rotates the joint, as in overarm swimming or tennis. More often they are very subtle: a slight click or jerk when the arm is raised above shoulder height, or the 'dead arm' sensation that overtakes the tennis player as he raises his racquet to serve.

Loss of function is expressed as inability to reach behind the back or difficulties with dressing and grooming.

EXAMINATION

While the patient gets undressed, observe how she moves, whether she can easily disengage her arms from the clothing, whether she can reach forwards, backwards and upwards, and whether or not she appears to be in pain.

Ensure that both shoulders, both arms, the chest and the neck are exposed. Ask the patient to stand where you can see her easily from in front, from behind and from the side. You may have to walk around her – or she may have to turn around – so that you can get the picture from all angles.

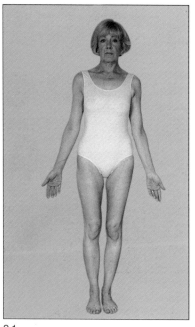

2.1

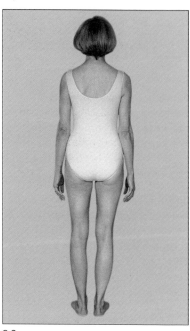

2.2

2.1 Stand back and look at the patient as a whole. Are the shoulders symmetrical and at the same level? Are the arms held in the same position on both sides, or is one arm persistently turned inwards or outwards? Compare the outlines of the clavicles, the acromioclavicular joints and the acromion prominences. Look for signs of muscle wasting: flattening of the deltoid bulge or the pectoral eminence.

2.2 Now stand behind the patient and follow the same routine, noting particularly the level of the shoulders, the position of the neck, the shape of the spine (is there scoliosis?) and the size and shape of the scapular outlines (is one scapula smaller, higher or more prominent than the other?). Again check for muscle wasting, particularly above the spine of the scapula on each side.

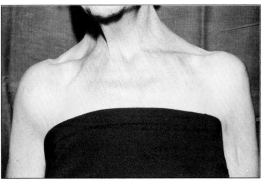

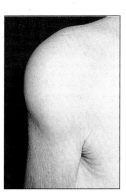

2.3

2.4

2.3, 2.4 Now come closer and look for old scars and local signs of swelling or inflammation. The patient in **2.3** has a swollen right shoulder, due to rheumatoid arthritis . The patient in **2.4** also has a 'swollen shoulder', but is it the joint? Or the muscle? Or the proximal end of the humerus? This proved to be a chondrosarcoma of the humerus.

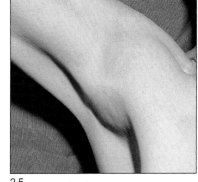

2.5

2.5 Don't forget to look in the axilla. A bulge may be produced by a large joint effusion, or by swollen lymph glands.

2.6 We're now ready to feel; for this the patient can be standing or sitting, and it's often easier to stand alongside the patient, with one hand tracing the bony outline while the other hand steers the arm into different positions. Start at the sternoclavicular joint, then move along the clavicle to the prominent acromioclavicular joint and the hard edge of the acromion process. Undue prominence and tenderness of the sternoclavicular or acromioclavicular joint may signify either malposition (subluxation) or arthritis.

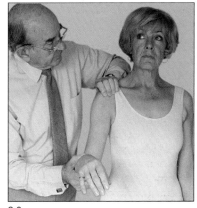

2.6

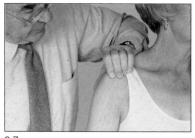

2.7

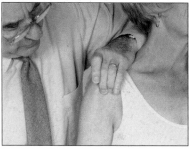

2.8

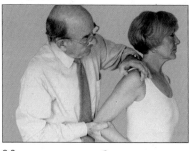

2.9

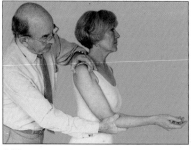

2.10

2.7 Try to localize any point of tenderness precisely. One of the commonest causes of shoulder pain is supraspinatus tendinitis. You can find the supraspinatus tendon by placing the tips of your fingers under the anterior edge of the acromion process.

2.8 The tendon of the long head of biceps is close by – a little lower than the supraspinatus, in the bicipital groove. You can find it quite easily by grasping the patient's elbow with one hand and turning the arm alternately into external and internal rotation; the tendon is felt slipping under your fingertips.

2.9, 2.10 A good test for supraspinatus tenderness is to place your middle finger firmly at the site of the tendon, under the anterior edge of the acromion, first with the shoulder in extension (this pushes the tendon forward against your finger and the patient flinches with pain) and then with the shoulder slightly flexed (now the tendon disappears under the overhang of the acromion process and the spot is no longer tender).

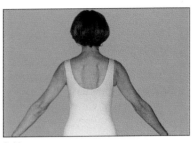

2.11

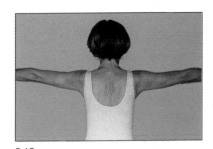

2.12

2.11–2.13 Movements are best observed from behind the patient, where you can also see the scapula. Start with abduction, noting not only the *range* of movement but also the *rhythm* and *symmetry* of movement; these features are the first to be disturbed in rotator cuff disorders. Ask the patient to raise her arms sideways and upwards above her head. This is normally carried out smoothly with co-ordination of the glenohumeral and the scapulothoracic components.

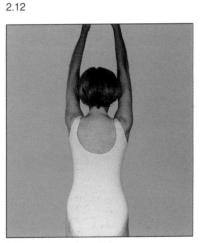

2.13

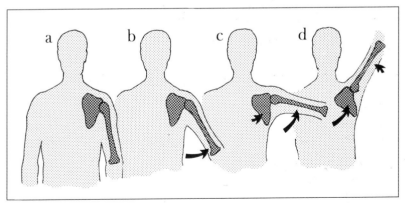

2.14

2.14 The first 90° of abduction takes place mainly at the glenohumeral joint. As the arm rises, the scapula begins to rotate on the thorax. In the last phase of abduction, movement is almost entirely scapulothoracic.

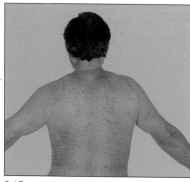

2.15

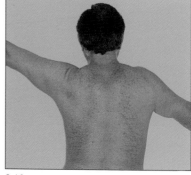

2.16

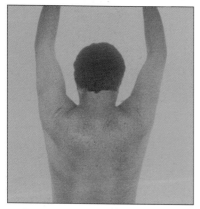

2.17

2.15–2.17 In this patient with supraspinatus tendinitis on theright side, the normal glenohumeral/scapulothoracic rhythm is disturbed. The scapula starts to move very early in abduction; between 100° and 120°, movement is painful and asymmetrical (the *'painful arc'*); beyond 120° the pain eases off and he can complete the full range of abduction.

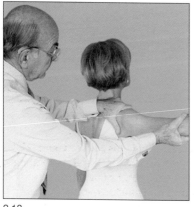

2.18

2.18 True glenohumeral movement occurs only up to 90°. It can be tested by isolating or fixing the scapula. This is done by pushing firmly down on the upper border of the scapula, thus preventing scapular rotation. Abduction now takes place only at the glenohumeral joint. A patient with a frozen shoulder may *appear* to be capable of abduction (because the scapula can still move) but this test will reveal the restriction of true glenohumeral movement.

2.19 Flexion and extension can be measured by asking the patient to lift the arms forwards and backwards as far as possible. The normal range is 0–170° for flexion and 0–40° for extension. This patient has limited extension of the left shoulder.

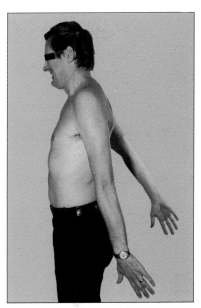

2.19

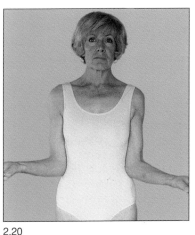

2.20

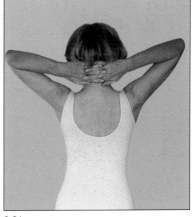

2.21

2.20, 2.21 External rotation is assessed first with the arms by the patient's sides and then with the arms abducted ('clasp your hands behind your neck'). Internal rotation in the anatomical position is hampered by the arms abutting against the body; you will gain a better idea of the range of movement by asking the patient to reach up behind her back and touch the scapula. By comparing the two sides, small differences can be detected (see **2.26** and **2.27**).

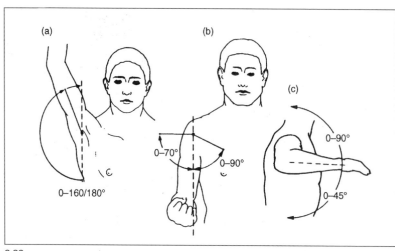

2.22

2.22 The normal ranges of movement are shown here. (a) Total abduction is from 0° to 160° (or even 180°), but only 90° of this movement takes place at the glenohumeral joint; the remainder is scapular movement. (b) With the arm lowered, external rotation is usually about 70°. (c) With the arm abducted to a right angle, external rotation is freer but internal rotation is somewhat restricted.

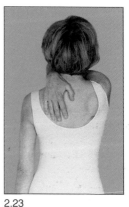 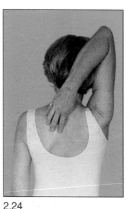 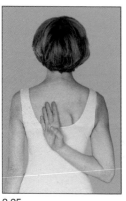

2.23   2.24   2.25

2.23–2.25 *The Apley scratch test.* Shoulder movement can be assessed very quickly by asking the patient to try and scratch an imaginary spot over the opposite scapula in three ways: by reaching over the opposite shoulder, by reaching behind the neck and by reaching behind her back. If she can do all three, think again about the source of pain.

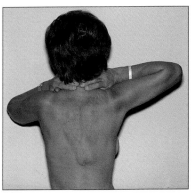

2.26

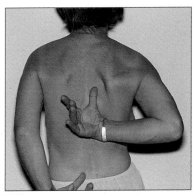

2.27

2.26, 2.27 This patient, who has a supraspinatus tendinitis (rotator cuff syndrome) on the left side, has restricted external and internal rotation; she obviously failed the scratch test.

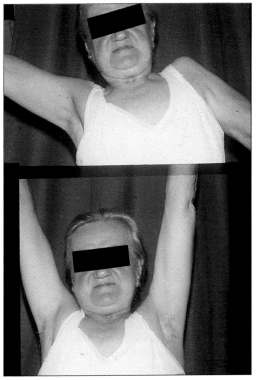

2.28

2.28 *The abductor paradox*. With a complete tear of the supraspinatus tendon, the patient cannot initiate abduction; however, once the arm is lifted passively, she can hold it abducted with her deltoid. The left side is abnormal in this patient.

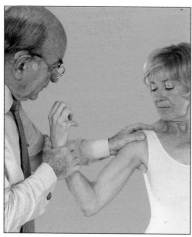

2.29

2.29 Testing for biceps function. When the patient flexes the elbow forcefully against resistance, the biceps stands out.

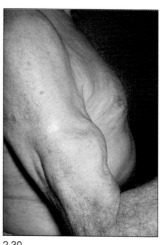

2.30

2.30 Ruptured biceps tendon. This elderly man tried to lift a slab of concrete and felt something snap. When he contracts his biceps, it bunches up into a ball in the front of his arm.

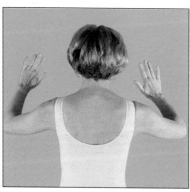

2.31

2.31 Testing for serratus anterior function. Ask the patient to push hard against the wall and compare the two sides. The scapulae are held flat against the rib-cage by the action of serratus anterior.

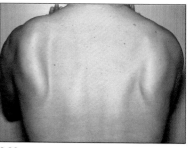

2.32

2.32 In serratus anterior palsy the patient cannot stabilize the scapula. This nurse developed brachial neuralgia (neuralgic amyotrophy) affecting the nerve to serratus anterior on the left. When she pushes against the wall, her left scapula lifts off the thorax; this is described as 'winging' of the scapula.

2.33 There are several ways of testing for stability of the shoulder joint. This is the *apprehension test* for anterior subluxation or dislocation. Abduct, externally rotate and extend the patient's shoulder, while pushing on the head of the humerus with the opposite thumb. If the patient feels that the joint is about to dislocate, she will forcibly (and volubly) resist the manoeuvre.

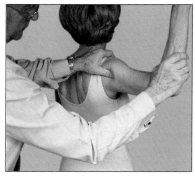

2.33

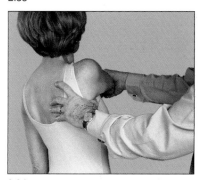

2.34

2.34 You can test for posterior instability in the same way by drawing the arm forward and across the body (adduction and internal rotation).

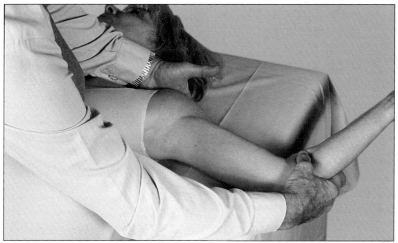

2.35

2.35 Doing the apprehension test with the patient lying down.

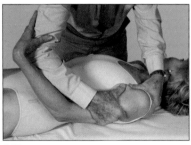 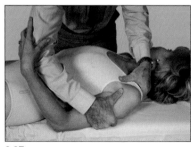

2.36   2.37

2.36, 2.37 If the shoulder is markedly unstable, you can passively move the head of the humerus backwards and forwards in and out of the glenoid fossa. Stabilize the scapula with one hand, grasp the patient's arm firmly with the other, and then alternately lift and push the humerus forwards and backwards. You can feel the joint subluxating.

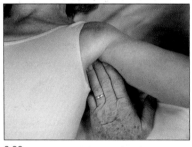

2.38

2.38 Lastly, don't forget to examine the axilla, the chest and the neck, any of which can be the source of unexplained shoulder pain.

THE ELBOW

3

HISTORY

Pain from the elbow joint is usually fairly diffuse and may extend into the forearm. Localized pain over the lateral or medial epicondyle of the humerus suggests a type of tendinitis – 'tennis elbow' or 'golfer's elbow'. Don't forget that 'elbow pain' may be referred from the neck!

Stiffness is hardly noticed if it is mild, but marked loss of movement is a considerable handicap. The patient may be unable to reach up to her mouth or hair, or down to her perineum. Limited pronation or supination interferes with carrying and holding activities.

Swelling may be due to injury or inflammation. Ask where the swelling is; a lump over the back of the elbow suggests an olecranon bursitis.

Deformity is uncommon except in rheumatoid arthritis and after trauma. Always ask about previous injuries.

Instability also occurs in rheumatoid arthritis and after trauma. The patient can feel the elbow jerking out of position when the muscles contract.

Neurological symptoms may be the main complaint. We have all experienced pain and tingling in the forearm or hand from a bump on the 'funny bone'. The same symptoms may occur with more persistence in elbow disorders which cause compression of or traction upon the ulnar nerve.

Loss of function is noticed in grooming activities, carrying, lifting and hand work. It has been said (and not facetiously) that the main functions of the elbow are to put food in the mouth and to cope with perineal hygiene.

EXAMINATION

While the patient undresses, notice how she uses her arms. Can she disengage from her clothes without difficulty?

Both upper limbs should be completely exposed, and it is essential to look at the back as well as the front. Often the neck, shoulders and hands also need to be examined.

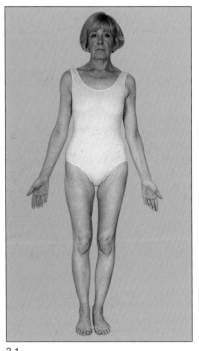

3.1

3.1 Begin by looking at the patient as a whole, taking in the neck and shoulders before concentrating on the elbows. Look at the skin, front and back. Are there any scars? Is the colour normal? Is there any swelling or deformity of the arms? Compare the position of the elbows with the arms turned out and the palms facing forward. Normally the elbows, when extended, are in 5–10° valgus; this is the normal carrying angle.

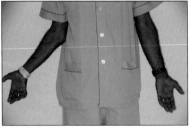

3.2

3.2 This man has excessive valgus of the right elbow. But his main complaint was of weakness and deformity in the hand, which was caused by traction on the ulnar nerve secondary to the elbow deformity.

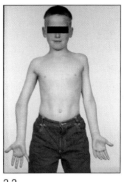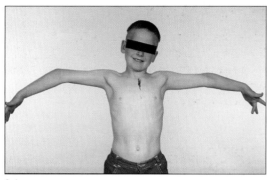

3.3   3.4

3.3, 3.4 This boy has a varus deformity of the right elbow, the sequel to a supracondylar fracture. It is even more obvious when he raises his arms. You can see why this is called a 'gunstock deformity'.

3.5 Localized swellings are often diagnostic. The enormous red lumps over the points of the elbows are enlarged olecranon bursae; the ruddy complexion completes the typical picture of gout.

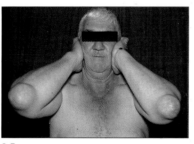

3.5

3.6 Feeling begins with the skin. Is there undue warmth? Next, feel the bony landmarks. With the elbow flexed, the tips of the medial and lateral epicondyles and the olecranon process form an isosceles triangle. With the elbow extended, they lie transversely in line with each other. These relationships are disturbed in post-traumatic deformities of the elbow.

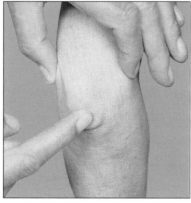

3.6

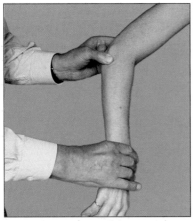

3.7

3.7 The lateral compartment of the elbow (the radio-humeral joint) is easily located; you can feel the head of the radius moving by placing your thumb a centimetre below the lateral epicondyle while your other hand pronates and supinates the forearm. The medial compartment cannot be accurately located.

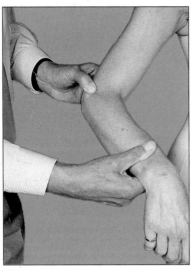

3.8

3.8 Tenderness just above the lateral epicondyle suggests a 'tennis elbow'. Of course the condition is not confined to tennis players; it is a tendinitis of the common extensor origin and it occurs most commonly in workers who use their wrist extensors in prolonged, repetitive tasks. (A similar condition on the medial side is called 'golfer's elbow').

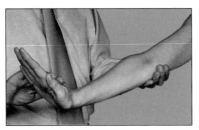

3.9

3.9 The pain of tennis elbow can be reproduced or intensified by active extension of the wrist against resistance (tension of the common extensor).

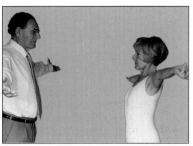 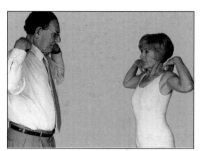

3.10   3.11

3.10, 3.11 The best way to examine active movements is to stand in front of the patient and show her what to do.

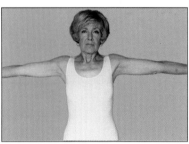 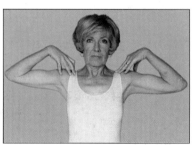

3.12   3.13

3.12, 3.13 The normal range of flexion is from 0° (full extension) to 140° (full flexion).

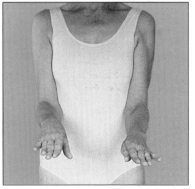 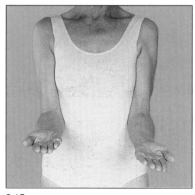

3.14   3.15

3.14, 3.15 To test pronation and supination, ask the patient to tuck her elbows tightly into her body and then turn the hands fully palms down and then palms up. The normal range is 90° in each direction.

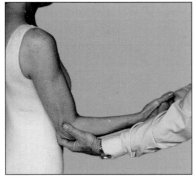

3.16

3.16 Tests for power and stability usually complete the examination. However, if the elbow is deformed, or if there is any other reason to suspect ulnar nerve tension or entrapment, you will also need to carry out a neurological examination of the hand.

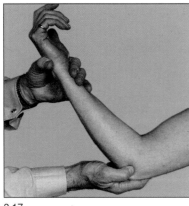

3.17

3.17 The ulnar nerve itself can be felt just behind the medial condyle. It may be thickened and unusually sensitive.

4

THE WRIST AND HAND

THE SETTING

The hand is, in more senses than one, the medium of introduction to the physical world. Deformity and loss of function are profoundly disabling and bitterly resented.

Pain may be sharply localized to one of the joints or tendons. Sometimes (as in rheumatoid arthritis) *all* the joints are painful. Pain which wakes the patient at night, but is slight or absent by day, may be due to a carpal tunnel syndrome. A poorly defined ache may be referred from the neck, shoulder or mediastinum.

Stiffness also may be confined to a particular joint, or it may be generalized. Early morning stiffness is typical of rheumatoid arthritis.

Locking or *snapping* of one finger is so characteristic that you can make the diagnosis on the history alone – tenovaginitis of the flexor tendon sheath. The finger gets stuck in partial flexion; then, with an effort, the patient overcomes the obstruction and the finger snaps out into full extension. The popular term *trigger finger* was probably inspired by watching too many movies!

Swelling around the wrist may signify involvement of either the joint or the tendon sheaths. Swelling (or swellings) of the fingers should make one think of arthritis. Characteristically rheumatoid arthritis affects the proximal joints and osteoarthritis the distal joints. Patients abhor knobbly fingers and may seek treatment chiefly for cosmetic reasons.

Deformity may appear suddenly (due to tendon rupture) or gradually (suggesting bone, joint or other pathology).

Loss of function is particularly troublesome in the hand. The patient may have difficulty handling eating utensils, holding a cup or glass, grasping a door knob or a crutch, dressing or (most trying of all) attending to personal hygiene. Loss of wrist function leads to weakness of grip.

Neurological symptoms include feelings of numbness and tingling, and motor weakness. The patient may complain of difficulty in doing up buttons, or sewing and writing, and in handling objects with safety and certainty.

EXAMINATION

Both upper limbs should be bared for comparison. Examination of the wrist and hand needs meticulous attention to detail. Always ask which is the dominant hand; you would expect it to be stronger and more adept. Patients who claim to be ambidextrous may turn out to be 'ambisinistrous'!

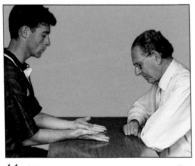

4.1

4.1 This is a good position for examination of the wrist and hand. Both you and the patient are sitting comfortably.

4.2

4.2 Begin with the palms upwards, noting any scars, abnormalities of colour, and callosities (the working man's hand). Is the skin dry or moist, normally wrinkled or smooth and atrophic? Take note of the resting posture, or attitude, of the hand; this may be an important clue to nerve or tendon damage.

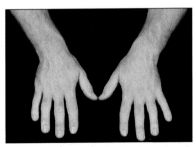

4.3

4.3 Then look at the back of the hands, again noting any signs of disuse (absence of hair and unusual smoothness). Is there pitting or scarring of the nails, a common feature of psoriasis?

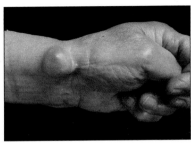

4.4

4.4 Swelling is usually quite obvious. Try to establish where it arises. This patient has a large ganglion arising from one of the tendon sheaths at the wrist; the rest of the hand is normal.

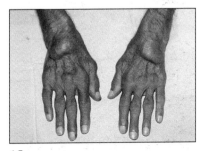

4.5

4.5 By contast, this patient has symmetrical swellings of the extensor tendon sheaths and all the proximal interphalangeal joints. This can only be rheumatoid arthritis.

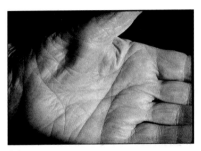

4.6

4.6 Wasting is often more difficult to detect. However, in this patient with a cut median nerve the thenar eminence is markedly flattened.

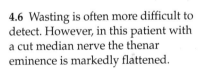

Deformities of the hand are often so typical that the diagnosis may be made at a glance. Learn to recognize them. A few of the more common disorders are illustrated here.

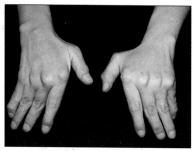

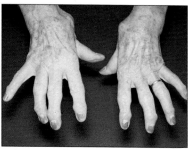

4.7

4.8

4.7, 4.8 The patient in **4.7** has symmetrical swelling and ulnar deviation of the *proximal* finger joints, particularly the metacarpo-phalangeal joints. This is typical of rheumatoid arthritis. The one in **4.8** has swelling and deformity of the *distal* joints. These are Heberden's nodes, the classical feature of polyarticular osteoarthritis; as is often the case in this condition, the thumb carpo-metacarpal joints also are affected.

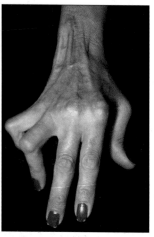

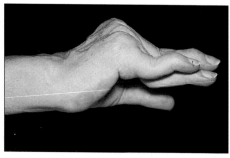

4.9

4.10

4.9, 4.10 The other common finger deformities in rheumatoid arthritis are *boutonnière* (**4.9**) and swan-neck (**4.10**).

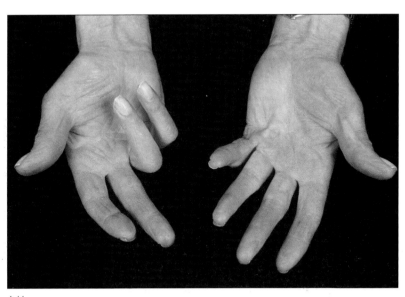

4.11

4.11 In Dupuytren's disease the finger deformities are produced by contracture of fibrous bands in the palmar fascia. There may also be firm fibrous nodules in the palm.

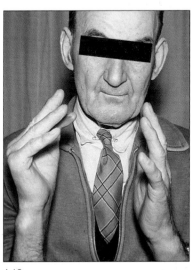

4.12 This man, too, has fixed flexion of the fingers in the right hand. He does not have arthritis and his palmar fascia is normal. These are ischaemic contractures of the intrinsic muscles secondary to a forearm compartment syndrome.

4.12

When feeling for tenderness, try to establish the site precisely. Knowing exactly where the tenderness is located is more than halfway to knowing what is causing it.

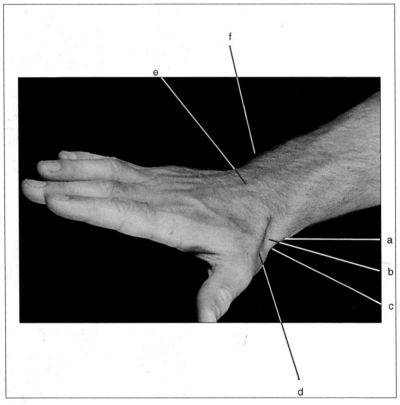

4.13

4.13 Before going on to feel, let us review a few points of surface anatomy. In this picture you can identify (a) the tip of the styloid process; (b) the anatomical snuffbox bounded on the radial side by (c) the extensor pollicis brevis and on the ulnar side by (d) the extensor pollicis longus; (e) the extensor tendons of the fingers; and (f) the head of the ulna.

4.14 Tenderness at the tip of the radial styloid suggests de Quervain's disease (tenovaginitis of the combined sheath for extensor pollicis brevis and abductor pollicis longus). This diagnosis can be confirmed by *Finkelstein's test*. Hold the patient's hand with his thumb tucked firmly into the palm; then turn the wrist into full ulnar deviation; in a positive test, this will elicit sharp pain in the affected sheath.

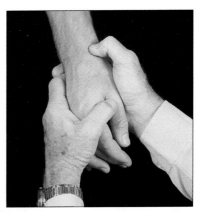

4.14

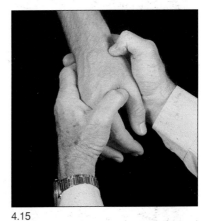

4.15 Tenderness in the anatomical snuffbox is typical of a scaphoid injury.

4.15

4.16 Tenderness just distal to the head of the ulna is found in extensor carpi ulnaris tendinitis.

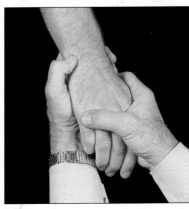

4.16

> *Now test movements of the wrist and hand - first active, then passive,
> then abnormal.*

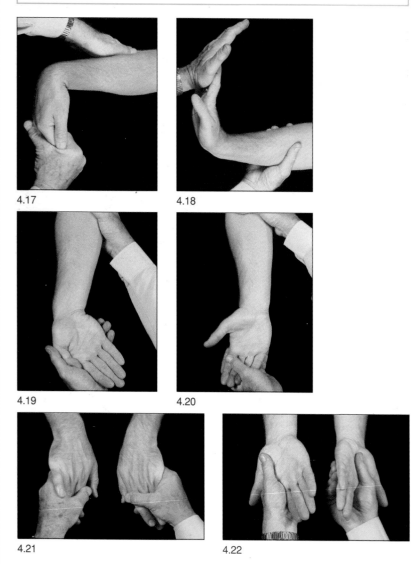

4.17

4.18

4.19

4.20

4.21

4.22

4.17–4.22 Testing for wrist flexion, extension, ulnar deviation, radial
deviation, pronation and supination. When testing pronation and supination,
the patient must keep his elbows flexed.

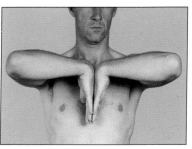

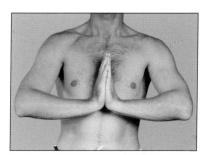

4.23   4.24

4.23, 4.24 This is a good way to test flexion and extension of the wrists; you can compare the two sides.

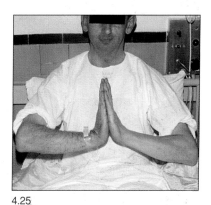

4.25 This patient has Kienböck's disease of the left wrist; extension is limited on that side.

4.25

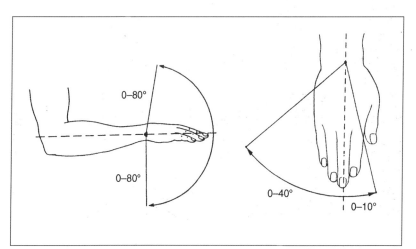

4.26

4.26 The normal ranges of movement at the wrist.

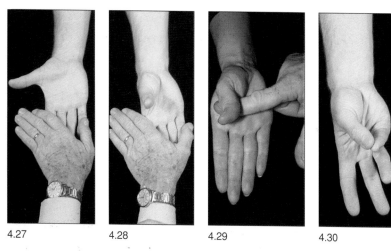

4.27   4.28   4.29   4.30

4.27–4.30 Testing for movements of the thumb. You should have no difficulty defining the planes of movement if you follow this routine: hold the patient's hand flat on the table and instruct him to 'stretch to the side' (extension), 'point to the ceiling' (abduction), 'pinch my finger' (adduction) and 'touch your little finger' (opposition).

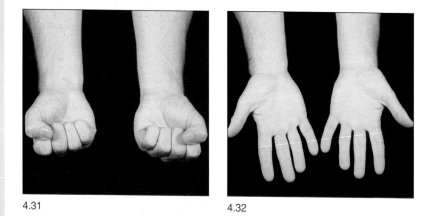

4.31   4.32

4.31, 4.32 Metacarpophalangeal and interphalangeal movements should be tested individually. Here, for the sake of brevity, we show the normal range from full flexion to full extension.

If active flexion of one finger is restricted, you will need to test whether the flexor tendons are intact.

4.33 To test flexor profundus, hold the proximal finger joint extended and ask the patient to bend the finger; if the tendon is intact, the distal phalanx will flex.

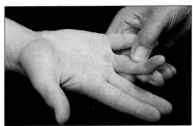

4.33

4.34 To test the flexor superficialis you must first inactivate the profundus. This is done by holding the other fingers extended; because the profundi act as one, you are now preventing profundus action also in the finger being tested. Any flexion must be due to superficialis action. If the finger cannot flex, the superficialis is not working.

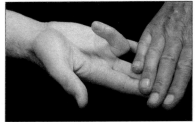

4.34

4.35, 4.36 In patients with arthritis, you may need to test for stability. This is done by grasping the finger firmly with one hand and shunting it backwards and forwards, as shown in this patient with rheumatoid disease.

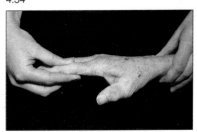

4.35

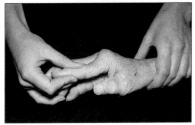

4.36

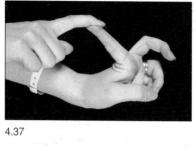

4.37

4.37 This young woman has generalized joint laxity; the fingers can hyperextend to beyond 90°, but the joints are stable.

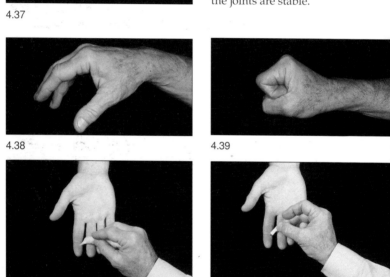

4.38

4.39

4.40

4.41

4.38–4.41 Neurological examination is important. Look at the posture of the hand, then test for grip strength, individual muscle power and sensibility to touch and pinprick.

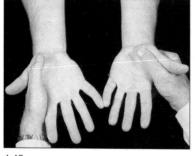

4.42

4.42 A good test for interosseous muscle function (ulnar nerve) is to have the patient spread his fingers apart (abduct) as strongly as possible; slowly push the hands together until the tips of the little fingers are forcefully opposing one another; the weaker one will collapse.

4.43 *Froment's test* is another way of comparing ulnar nerve function in the two hands. Ask the patient to grip a card firmly between thumbs and index fingers; the thumb adductors are brought forcefully into play. If the adductor pollicis is weak, the patient can hold on to the card only by acutely flexing the interphalangeal joint of the thumb (flexor pollicis longus is supplied by the median nerve).

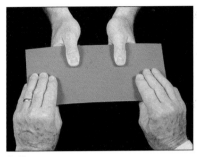

4.43

4.44–4.46 This patient has a high ulnar nerve injury on the right. There is mild clawing of the fourth and fifth fingers (**4.44**); she has weakness of the finger abductors (**4.45**); and Froment's test is positive (compare **4.46** and **4.43**).

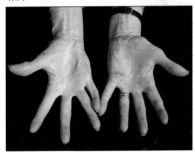

4.44

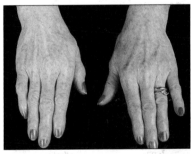

4.45

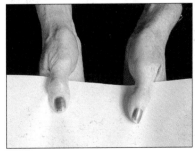

4.46

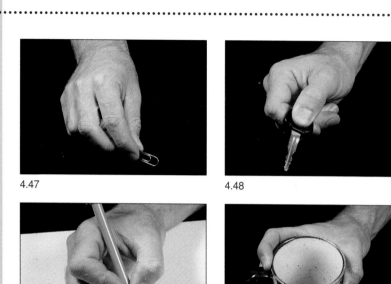

4.47

4.48

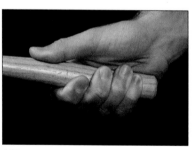

4.49

4.50

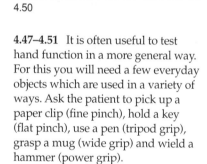

4.51

4.47–4.51 It is often useful to test hand function in a more general way. For this you will need a few everyday objects which are used in a variety of ways. Ask the patient to pick up a paper clip (fine pinch), hold a key (flat pinch), use a pen (tripod grip), grasp a mug (wide grip) and wield a hammer (power grip).

5

THE NECK

HISTORY

Pain in the neck may start suddenly (as with an acute intervertebral disc prolapse) or gradually (as in chronic disc degeneration and osteo-arthritis). By far the commonest cause of neck-ache is a simple postural strain. Typically the pain is felt at the back of the neck, but it may radiate upwards to the occiput or across to the shoulder(s) or arm(s). Always ask if the patient injured his neck at any time in the past.

Stiffness often accompanies pain; indeed, pain may give rise to stiffness because of muscle spasm. Progressively severe stiffness signifies some-thing more – usually chronic disc degeneration or arthritis of the facet joints.

Deformity usually appears as a wry neck, or as fixed flexion. If it is of recent onset and accompanied by pain, think of a prolapsed inter-vertebral disc.

Neurological symptoms, such as numbness, tingling or weakness in the arm(s) or hand(s), suggest compression or irritation of a nerve root. Weakness of the lower limbs may result from cord damage.

'Whiplash syndrome' is the rather bizarre name given to a group of symptoms which often follows a jerking strain such as might occur in a motor car collision. It comprises any number of the following: neck pain, paraesthesia, headache, dizziness, tinnitus, dysphagia and inter-mittent blurring of vision.

EXAMINATION

Pay attention to the patient's posture and the ease, or difficulty, with which he turns his head from side to side while he undresses. Is he wearing a surgical collar?

The entire upper trunk and both upper limbs should be exposed. Start with the patient standing, and be prepared to move around so that you can approach him from the front, the back or either side.

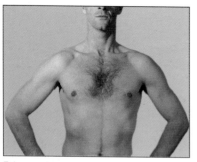

5.1

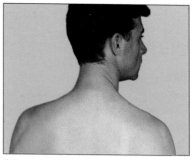

5.2

5.1, 5.2 Look at the patient as a whole. Are the outlines of the neck and shoulders symmetrical? Is there muscle wasting, or muscle spasm, either in front or at the back of the neck? Are there scars? A 'necklace scar' (an anterior transverse scar in the line of the skinfolds) may be almost invisible.

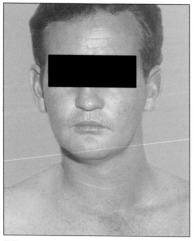

5.3

5.3 Is the position of the neck normal, or is it skew? This patient has a mild but definite wry neck, due to a prolapsed intervertebral disc.

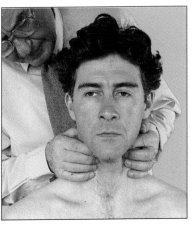
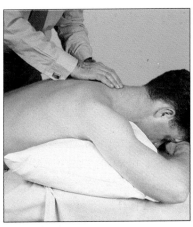

5.4   5.5

5.4, 5.5 The front of the neck is best felt with the patient seated and the examiner standing behind him. The back of the neck is more reliably felt with the patient lying prone and resting his head over a pillow. In this way muscle spasm is reduced and the structures at the back of the neck are better defined. Feel each of the posterior spinous processes. Are they evenly spaced? Is there tenderness in the midline? Now move your fingers down the neck a thumb's breadth from the midline. This marks the line of the facet joints, although they cannot be individually defined. But is there tenderness at any level? Then gently explore the soft-tissues in the supraclavicular and suprascapular regions. 'Referred' muscle tenderness is common in almost all chronic cervical spine disorders.

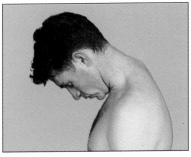
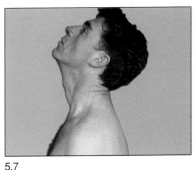

5.6   5.7

5.6, 5.7 Now examine the neck for range of movement in all directions. This is best observed as assisted active movement. Ask the patient to move and then help the movement on to its maximum without hurting the patient. Start with flexion ('chin on chest'), then extension ('look up at the ceiling').

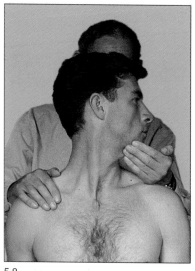 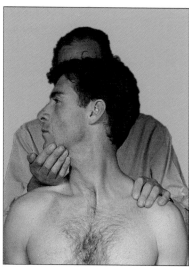

5.8   5.9

5.8, 5.9 Similarly with rotation to each side in turn ('look over your shoulder').

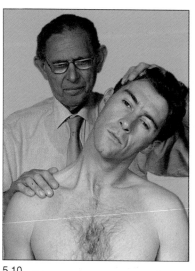 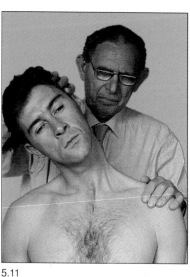

5.10   5.11

5.10, 5.11 Then lateral flexion to the left and to the right ('put your ear on your shoulder').

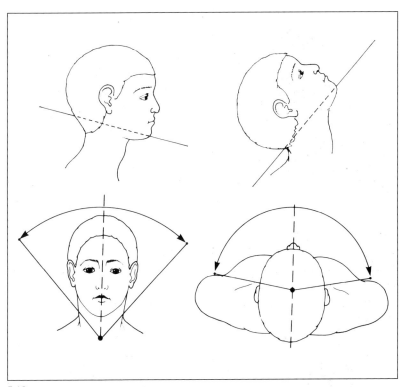

5.12

5.12 The normal ranges are shown. In full flexion the chin should touch the chest; in full extension the imaginary line joining the chin to the posterior occipital protuberance (the occipito-mental line) forms an angle of at least 45° with the horizontal and usually over 60° in young people. Lateral flexion and rotation are equal in both directions.

Neurological assessment is an essential part of the examination of the neck. With the patient standing or sitting you can test for power of shoulder abduction (C5, 6) and serratus anterior (C5, 6, 7) (see Chapter 2). The rest of the neurological examination is performed with the patient lying down.

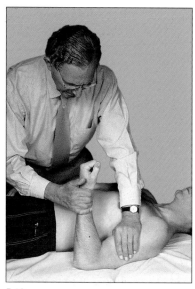
5.13

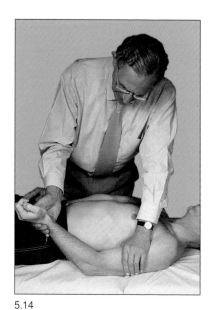
5.14

5.13, 5.14 Test for power of elbow flexion (C5, 6) and extension (C6, 7).

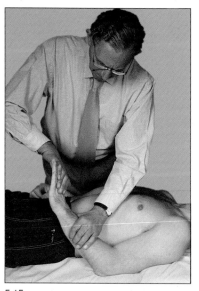
5.15

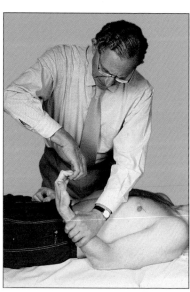
5.16

5.15, 5.16 Then wrist extension (C6, 7) and flexion (C7, 8).

5.17 The intrinsic muscles of the hand are supplied by C8 and T1. A useful way of testing the strength of finger abduction is to ask the patient to spread his fingers as strongly as possible, then take his hands in your own and force the little fingers together; the weaker side will give way.

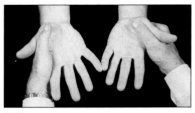

5.17

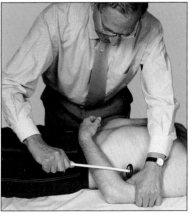

5.18

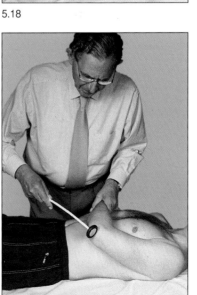

5.20

5.19

5.18–5.20 Tendon reflexes are tested at the biceps (C5, 6), the brachioradialis (C6) and the triceps (C7).

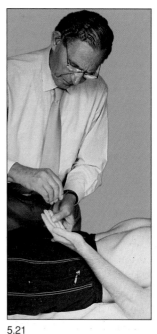

5.21

5.21 Sensibility to touch and pinprick should be carefully assessed and any abnormal areas mapped out.

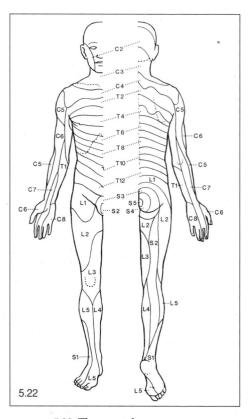

5.22

5.22 The normal sensory areas (dermatomes).

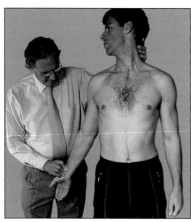

5.23

5.23 If a thoracic outlet syndrome is suspected, the vascular status should be assessed. In *Adson's test* the radial pulse is felt while the arm is slightly abducted, extended and externally rotated; then ask the patient to take a deep breath and turn his head to the side being tested. If the pulse disappears it suggests that the subclavian artery is being compressed by a bony or soft-tissue obstruction at the thoracic outlet.

6

THE BACK

HISTORY

Pain is the usual presenting symptom. It may start suddenly, perhaps after a lifting strain, or it may come on gradually. Backache is usually felt low down at the lumbosacral junction, but it often extends to one or other side of the midline and into the upper part of the buttock.

'Sciatica' is pain radiating from the buttock into the thigh and calf. It seems to follow the distribution of the sciatic nerve (hence the name), but it is not necessarily caused by nerve pathology. More often than not it is *referred pain* from some other structure – usually one of the vertebral joints. However, if it is regularly aggravated by coughing or straining, and even more so if it is accompanied by numbness or tingling in the leg, it probably arises from one of the lumbo-sacral nerve roots.

Stiffness may be sudden in onset and almost complete (after a disc prolapse) or continuous and predictably worse in the mornings (suggesting arthritis or ankylosing spondylitis).

Deformity may take the form of a 'skew back', due to muscle spasm, or it may signify a true structural abnormality, e.g. scoliosis or excessive kyphosis.

Neurological symptoms may not at first be associated, in the patient's mind, with a back problem. Ask specifically about feelings of numbness or tingling, or possibly weakness, in the lower limbs. The exact distribution is important and will help to pinpoint the site of pathology.

Urinary retention or incontinence may be due to pressure on the cauda equina. Always enquire about this – it may signal the need for urgent treatment.

Other symptoms, which the patient may fail to mention, are *urethral discharge, diarrhoea* and *sore eyes* – features associated with Reiter's disease and spondylitis.

EXAMINATION

By the time the patient is ready to be examined, you would have noticed his gait and posture, how he rises from his chair and how easily he is able to undress.

The trunk and both lower limbs should be exposed. The examination proceeds in three stages: with the patient first upright, then lying face downwards and then lying face upwards.

With the patient upright

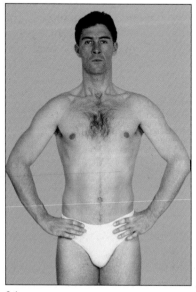

6.1 Stand face to face with your patient and look at his physique and posture. Are the two sides of his body completely symmetrical? Does he have any scars or blemishes on his chest or abdomen? Is there any wasting of his thighs?

6.1

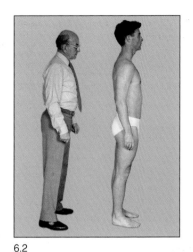

6.2

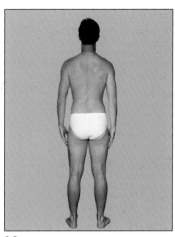

6.3

6.2, 6.3 Now move around and stand behind the patient. Look at his general posture and shape. Does he stand upright, or does he lean over to one side? Is the pelvis level, or is one leg shorter than the other? Is there excessive curvature of the thoracic spine (hyperkyphosis), or hollowing of the lumbar spine (hyperlordosis)? Does he have any lateral curvature (scoliosis)? Now look carefully for scars or other skin markings that may suggest a spinal disorder. Take note of any lumps or muscle spasm.

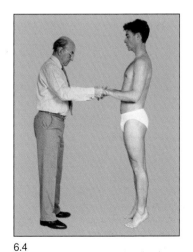

6.4

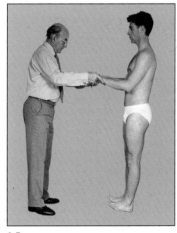

6.5

6.4, 6.5 Ask him to stand on his toes, then on his heels. Next, to walk a few paces, first on his toes, then on his heels. If he can do all, he must have good balance and muscle power in plantarflexion and dorsiflexion of the ankles.

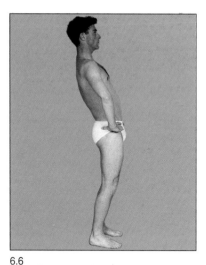

6.6

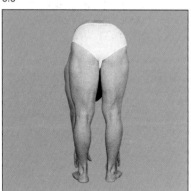

6.7

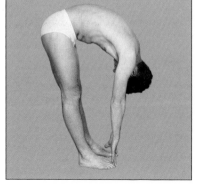

6.8

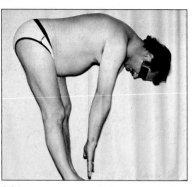

6.9

6.6 Standing behind the patient, examine movements of the spine. Begin with extension, by asking him to lean backwards. If he has back pain, he will find this easier than bending forward. Look at our model; his knees should be straight, otherwise you may be misled.

6.7–6.9 The normal range of flexion varies considerably; most people can reach only to their shins with the knees held straight. What is more important is the way the patient moves. His back should bend forward rhythmically, making a gentle arc from pelvis to shoulders (**6.8**). Compare the patient in **6.9**. He can bend over to touch his toes, but his lumbar spine is completely flat and ankylosed; all the 'flexion' is in his hips.

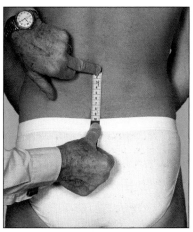
6.10

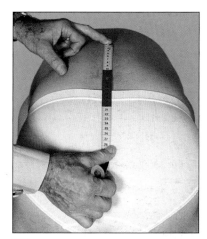
6.11

6.10, 6.11 You can measure the lumbar excursion. With the patient upright, select two bony points 10cm apart and mark the skin; as the patient bends forward, the two points should separate by at least a further 5cm.

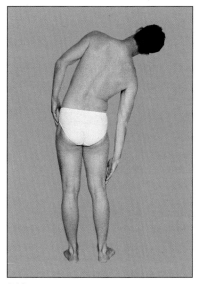
6.12

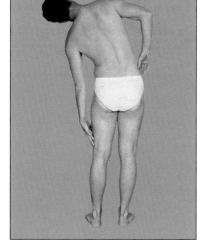
6.13

6.12, 6.13 Lateral flexion is tested by asking the patient to bend sideways, sliding his hand down the outer side of his leg; the two sides are compared.

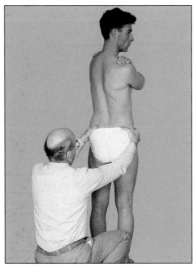

6.14

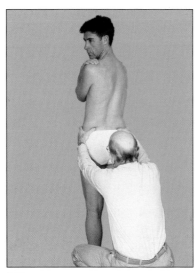

6.15

6.14, 6.15 To test rotation, anchor the pelvis in the neutral position and ask the patient to twist first to one side and then to the other. This movement takes place mainly in the thoracic spine and it should therefore not be restricted in lumbosacral disease.

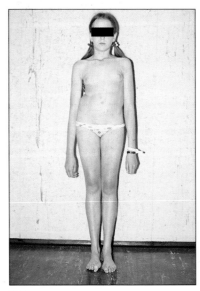

6.16

6.16 The diagnosis can often be made by merely looking and testing movements. This young girl complained mainly of having difficulty fitting clothes. She has an abnormal posture: the left shoulder is higher than the right and the right 'hip' is more prominent than the left.

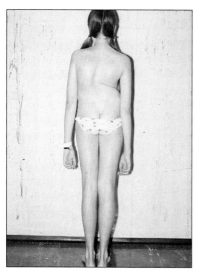

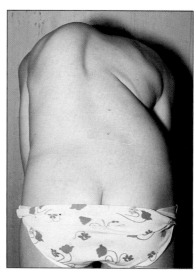

6.17

6.18

6.17, 6.18 The back view shows that she has a marked scoliosis. The rib hump becomes more prominent when she bends forward (**6.18**).

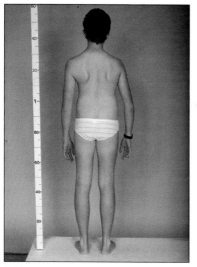

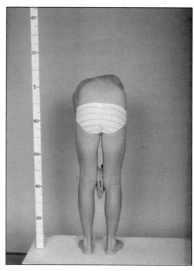

6.19

6.20

6.19, 6.20 Minor curves may become apparent only when the spine is flexed; note the asymmetry and the slight hump in **6.20**. Purely postural curves disappear when the patient flexes.

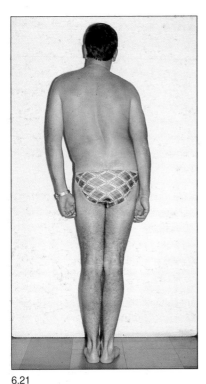

6.21

6.21 This is a postural curve. It is due to spasm of the paravertebral muscles following a disc prolapse.

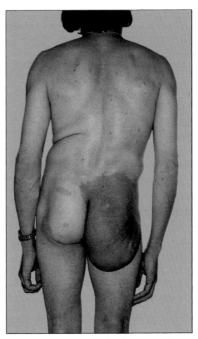

6.22

6.22 This patient has a structural curve plus multiple skin lesions. The diagnosis: neurofibromatosis.

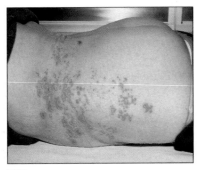

6.23

6.23 Always expect the unexpected. This woman had acute 'back pain' and 'sciatica'. After a cursory examination, her doctor said 'It's probably a disc'. Had he looked more closely, he would have spotted the tiny herpetiform rash. After two more weeks of torment, the rash is now glaringly obvious. The diagnosis: herpes zoster ('shingles').

With the patient prone

6.24 Observe how the patient gets onto the couch. Does he manage this easily or are there lots of grunts and groans? Make sure that he is lying comfortably and that he is relaxed; remove the pillow, so that he is not forced to arch his back. You can now see more clearly the backs of his thighs and legs. Check for gluteal wasting. Then gently feel along the spinous processes for any local bump (kyphos) or step in the vertebral column. Repeat the process three finger-breadths from the midline on each side, the line of the articular processes and the facet joints. Note the site of any unusual tenderness.

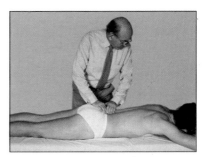

6.24

6.25 *Femoral stretch test.* This test is performed to detect undue irritability or tension of the nerve roots supplying the femoral nerve (L2, 3, 4). With the hip extended, the femoral nerve can be 'stretched' by passively flexing the knee; in a positive test, the patient complains of acute pain in the front of the thigh.

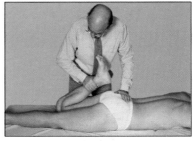

6.25

6.26 A 'false positive' may be due to tightness of the quadriceps. The test should be repeated with the knee held straight and the hip pulled into hyperextension.

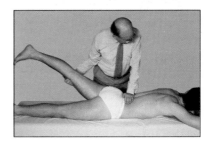

6.26

6.27 Pain is markedly increased when the previous two manoeuvres are combined.

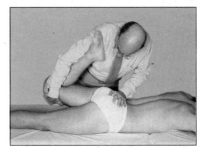

6.27

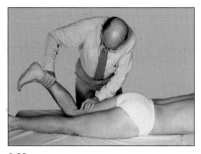

6.28

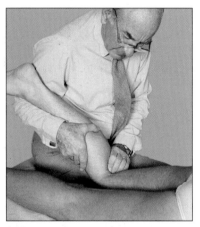

6.29

6.28 While the patient is lying prone, take the opportunity to test those muscles (the glutei and hamstrings in particular) which are difficult to examine with the patient supine. Hamstring power (L4, 5) is tested by asking him to flex the knee against resistance; your free hand can palpate the individual tendons at the back of the knee. Gluteus maximus power is tested by having the patient squeeze the buttocks together while you feel for muscle bulk and firmness on each side. An important part of the neurological examination (sadly, often omitted) is to test for skin sensation in the 'saddle' area (S3, 4 over and between the buttocks) and for the anal reflex (S4, 5). This is obligatory in patients with suspected cauda equina symptoms.

6.29, 6.30 The 'prone' examination is completed by feeling the popliteal and tibial pulses.

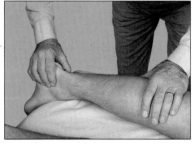

6.30

With the patient supine

Ask the patient to turn onto his back and observe how he does so. This may provide further clues to the diagnosis and the degree of functional loss.

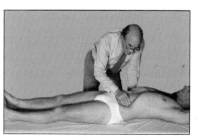

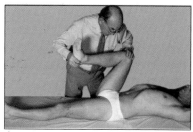

6.31

6.32

6.31, 6.32 Make him comfortable, and then examine the abdomen and the hips to exclude any abnormality in these areas. Compare the limbs for muscle wasting.

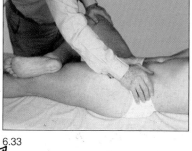

6.33 *Testing the sacroiliac joint.* It is very difficult to stress the sacroiliac joint as an isolated entity, and many people doubt that this can yield any useful information. One test for sacroiliac pain is the so-called *FABER manoeuvre* (**f**lexion, **ab**duction, **e**xternal **r**otation). The position of the leg is shown in **6.33**. Now press firmly down on the knee. Pain in the groin suggests a hip problem; pain in the back is said to indicate sacroiliac dysfunction.

6.33

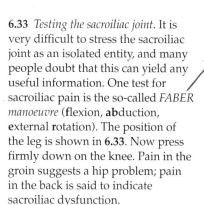

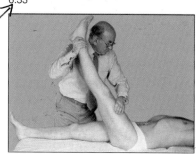

6.34

6.34 *Sciatic stretch tests.* In patients who complain of sciatica, it is important to determine whether 'stretching' the sciatic nerve reproduces or aggravates the pain; this will help to tell whether the nerve roots supplying the sciatic nerve are under tension. The simplest of these tests is the *straight-leg raising test.* While ensuring that the knee remains absolutely straight, lift the leg slowly until the patient stops you. Normally the leg can be raised to 80° or 90° without eliciting pain or resistance. In a positive test – for example after a disc prolapse – the patient experiences intense pain in the back of the thigh and buttock at less than 60°.

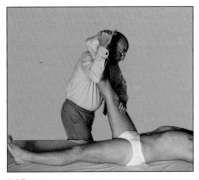

6.35

6.35 Straight-leg raising is sometimes combined with passive dorsiflexion of the ankle (*Lasegue's test*). This markedly aggravates the 'sciatic' pain.

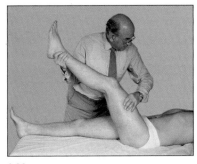

6.36

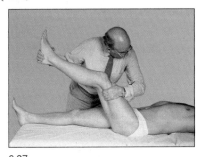

6.37

6.36, 6.37 This is a confirmatory test for sciatic tension. Repeat the straight-leg raise. At the point where the patient experiences pain, relax the nerve and the hamstring muscles by bending the knee slightly (**6.36**); the pain disappears. Now, with your free hand, press very firmly behind the lateral hamstrings so as to 'bowstring' the underlying common peroneal nerve (**6.37**); the pain recurs with renewed intensity.

Neurological examination is essential in all patients with back symptoms. This was begun when the patient was standing (walking on toes and heels) and was taken up again when he was prone. The examination is completed with the patient supine.

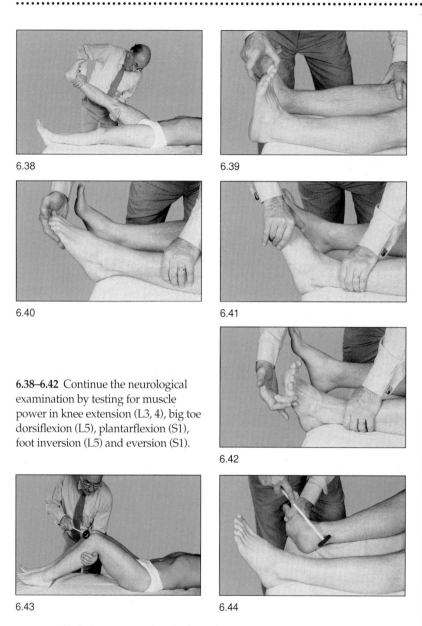

6.38

6.39

6.40

6.41

6.38–6.42 Continue the neurological examination by testing for muscle power in knee extension (L3, 4), big toe dorsiflexion (L5), plantarflexion (S1), foot inversion (L5) and eversion (S1).

6.42

6.43

6.44

6.43, 6.44 Reflexes are tested at the knee (L3, 4) and the ankle (S1). There is no direct reflex test for L5. However, if the knee jerk on one side is unusually brisk, this may signify weakness of the antagonist muscles – the knee flexors – which are supplied by L5.

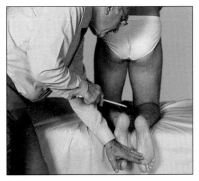

6.45

6.45 If you are doubtful about the ankle jerks, this is a good method for comparing the two sides. The patient kneels with the feet close together. Hold the ankles at right angles and tap the heel tendon of each ankle in quick succession. Small differences in briskness of response are readily detected.

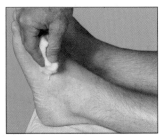

6.46

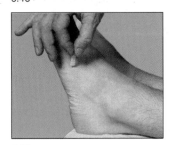

6.47

6.46, 6.47 The examination ends with a careful assessment of sensibility to touch and pinprick.

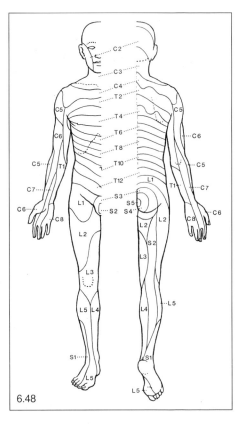

6.48

6.48 The normal dermatomes.

THE HIP

7

HISTORY

Pain arising in the hip is characteristically felt in the groin and the front of the thigh. However, it is often referred to the knee, and in some cases knee pain is the only symptom! Pain at the back of the hip is seldom from the joint; it usually derives from the lumbar spine. If an athlete or footballer complains of pain deep in the groin, think of a strain disorder (adductor tendinitis, traumatic osteitis pubis) or even a stress fracture.

Limp is the next most common symptom. It may simply be a way of coping with pain, but it could have other connotations such as a change in limb length, weakness of the hip abductors or instability.

Snapping or clicking in the hip may be due to a number of causes, including slipping of the gluteus maximus tendon backwards and forwards over the edge of the greater trochanter, a psoas bursitis, or (more rarely) detachment of the acetabular labrum. The patient may say that the hip 'slips out of joint', but this is seldom if ever the case.

Stiffness and *deformity* are late symptoms of hip disorder. Because pelvic mobility is able to compensate quite well for loss of hip movement, patients are unaware of small changes in the range of motion.

Functional activity may be progressively curtailed. Walking becomes slower and more tiresome; stairs are difficult to negotiate; sitting down and standing up become a burden; putting on socks and shoes is difficult; walking distance is curtailed; or, reluctantly, the patient starts using a walking stick.

EXAMINATION

As soon as the patient appears you will notice whether she limps or uses a walking stick, and whether she is in pain. For the formal examination, both lower limbs should be completely exposed from groin to toes. The examination proceeds in three stages: with the patient upright, then sitting and then lying.

With the patient upright

There should be enough space to examine the patient from all angles and to see how she walks.

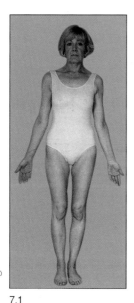

7.1

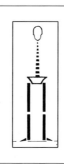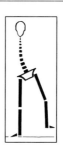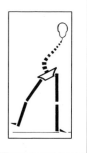

7.2

7.1 Stand back and look at her posture. Are the lower limbs symmetrical, or is one limb shorter or thinner than the other? Is the pelvis level and the spine quite straight? Are there any scars or swellings?

7.2 *Trendelenburg's sign.* This is a test for postural stability when the patient stands on one leg. The principle is illustrated in this figure. (a) In normal two-legged stance the body's centre of gravity is placed midway between the two feet. (b) Normally, in one-legged stance, the pelvis is pulled up on the unsupported side and the centre of gravity is placed directly over the standing foot. (c) If the weightbearing hip is unstable, the pelvis *drops* on the unsupported side; to avoid falling, the person has to throw his body towards the loaded side so that the centre of gravity is again over that foot.

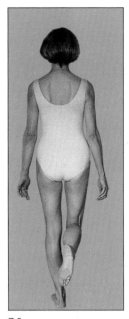

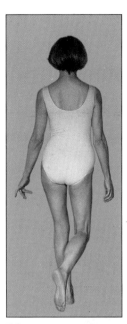

7.3

7.4

7.3, 7.4 Ask your patient to lift one leg, flexing the knee but not the hip. Normally the buttock-fold will rise on the unsupported side. In **7.4** our model is simulating a positive Trendelenburg sign; the buttock-fold drops on the unsupported side.

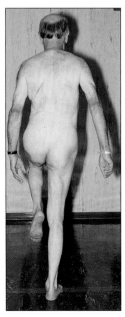

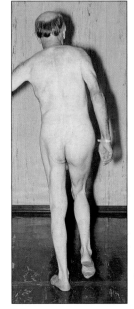

7.5

7.6

7.5, 7.6 Here is a patient with a genuine positive Trendelenburg sign on the left side. He has osteoarthritis. It is not usually necessary to have the patient completely undressed; we have done so in this case only to demonstrate a particular feature.

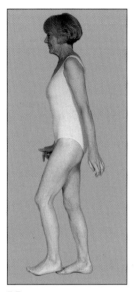
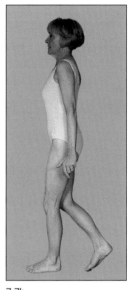
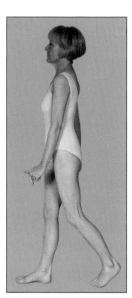

7.7a   7.7b   7.7c

7.7a,b,c *Gait*. Ask the patient to walk and observe, in turn, each phase of her gait – first by looking at general features such as rhythm and speed, then by concentrating on one limb at a time as it moves from heel-strike to stance to push-off and swing. The commonest abnormalities are a *short-leg limp* (a regular, even dip on the short side), an *antalgic gait* (an irregular limp, with the patient moving off the painful side as quickly as possible); and a *Trendelenburg lurch* – a variant of Trendelenburg's sign; the patient throws her body towards the affected side to avoid collapsing on a painful, weak or unstable hip.

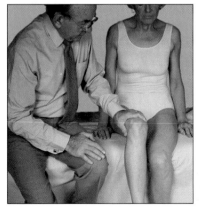

7.8

With the patient sitting

7.8 *Testing iliopsoas function*. This is best done with the patient sitting. Ask her to lift the thigh (flex the hip) against resistance. In this position the psoas is acting while the other hip flexors are relaxed. Pain or weakness suggests a local disorder such as a psoas bursitis.

With the patient lying down

Notice how the patient gets onto the examination couch, and whether she appears to be in pain.

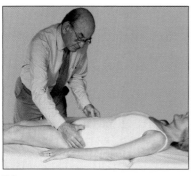

7.9

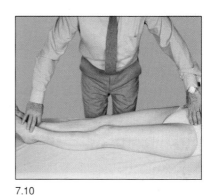

7.10

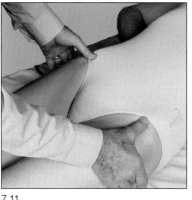

7.11

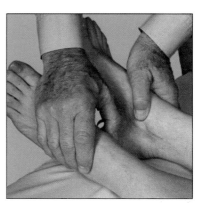

7.12

7.9–7.12 Make sure that she is lying comfortably; check that the pelvis is horizontal (both anterior superior iliac spines (ASIS) at the same level) and the legs placed symmetrically. Are the medial malleoli at the same level (i.e. is leg length equal)? Look for scars or sinuses, swelling or wasting anywhere from hip to toe. Note the position which the patient naturally adopts; is one limb rotated outwards or inwards?

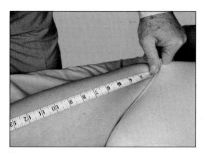

7.13

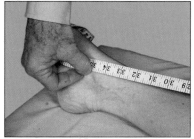

7.14

7.13, 7.14 Measuring is more precise; and technique is important. The limbs should be placed in identical positions. Hold the tape hard up against a fixed bony point (the ASIS in **7.13**) and run it straight to a distal bony landmark (the tip of the medial malleolus in **7.14**).

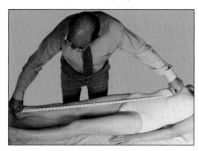

7.15

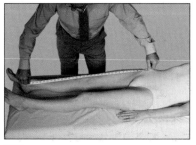

7.16

7.15, 7.16 Take two measurements on each side: one from the xiphisternum to the medial malleolus, the *'apparent length'* (**7.15**), and one from the ASIS to the malleolus, the *'real length'*, (**7.16**). A discrepancy in *apparent length* could be due either to a true difference in leg length or to lateral tilting of the pelvis (you can easily make your own leg 'shorter' or 'longer' by hitching your pelvis up on one side).
A discrepancy in *real length* may be due to shortening (or lengthening) of either the tibia or the femur, or both.

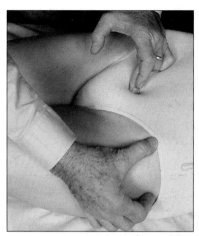

7.17 Feel for the landmarks that will tell you whether the hip is in its normal position and that will allow you to localize points of tenderness. Here the examiner's left middle finger is on the symphysis pubis, his right thumb is on the ASIS; the inguinal ligament stretches between these two points.

7.17

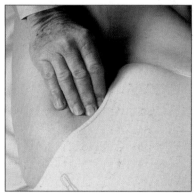

7.18

7.18 Half-way along the line of the inguinal ligament you can feel the femoral pulse; deep to this point is the femoral head.

7.19 Now use both hands to compare the two sides. Place each thumb on the ASIS and, with your middle finger, find the tip of the greater trochanter on each side. You will be aware of any asymmetry; if one greater trochanter is higher than the other, that hip is probably abnormal.

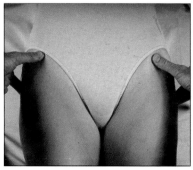

7.19

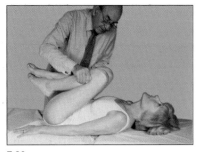

7.20

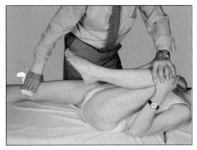

7.21

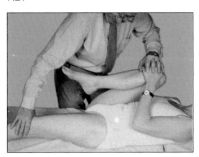

7.22

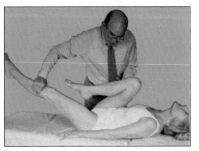

7.23

7.20–7.22 When testing movement, you have to be sure it is the hip, and not the pelvis, which is moving. To do this, you can use one limb to fix the pelvis while you measure the range of movement in the opposite hip. Flex both hips as far as they will go, noting the angle on each side (**7.20**). Then, with the patient's help, hold the left side fully flexed so as to stop the pelvis from rotating, while you lower the right leg as far as it will go (**7.21**). Change hands and repeat the manoeuvre to give you the range of movement on the left side.

7.23 *Thomas' test*. If the pelvis is not fixed during flexion and extension, the patient can easily overcome any limitation in movement by tilting the pelvis forwards and backwards. Thus, even a severe fixed flexion deformity can be completely masked simply by arching the back into hyperlordosis and tilting the pelvis. The 'deception' is unmasked by examining flexion and extension as described above. Our model is simulating a fixed flexion deformity on the left side. With the right hip fully flexed so as to stabilize the pelvis and straighten out the lumbar spine, the left hip cannot extend to zero. Thomas' test has revealed a fixed flexion deformity of 30°. Fixed flexion and loss of movement are common in osteoarthritis.

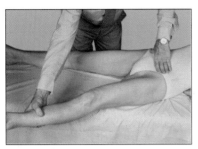

7.24

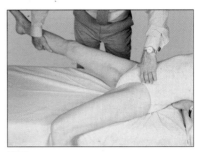

7.25

7.24, 7.25 The same principle is applied in measuring the range of abduction. First spread the legs as far as they will go, making sure that the pelvis is horizontal. Then drop the left leg (or the heel) over the edge of the couch in order to fix the pelvis in this position while you measure the range of abduction on the right side. Your left hand ensures that the pelvis stays horizontal.

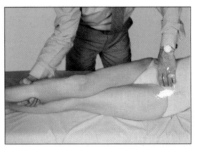

7.26

7.26 For testing adduction, you cannot really fix the pelvis. However, by spreading the fingers of your left hand between the ASISs, or by simply placing one hand firmly on the ilium, you can tell when the pelvis starts to rock as you adduct the leg.

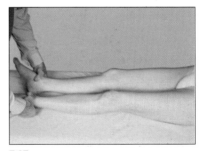

7.27

7.27, 7.28 To test rotation, stand at the foot of the couch; grasp both ankles firmly and twist the legs outwards (external rotation) and then inwards (internal rotation). Watch the knees, not the feet, to see how far the hips have rotated.

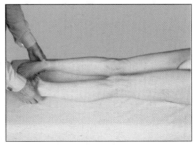

7.28

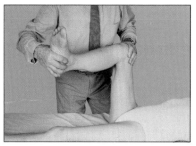

7.29

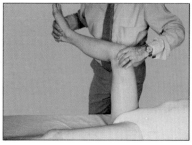

7.30

7.29, 7.30 Repeat the test for rotation with the hip and knee held in 90° flexion. Compare the two sides (**7.29** is external rotation and **7.30** is internal rotation of the hip).

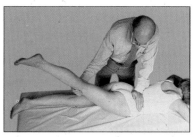

7.31

7.31 Lastly, ask the patient to roll over into the prone position. Check for scars or sinuses. Feel for tenderness and test the range of hip extension.

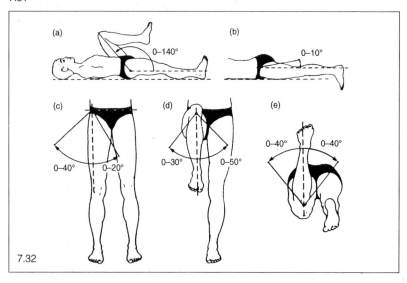

7.32

7.32 The normal ranges of movement at the hip.

8

THE KNEE

HISTORY

Pain is the most common knee symptom. With inflammatory or degenerative disorders it is usually diffuse; with mechanical disorders, and especially after injury, it is often localized – the patient can, and should, point to the painful spot. Young people often complain of *anterior knee pain*. This is pain around the patella, especially after strenuous activity or on going down stairs; not surprisingly it usually turns out to be due to some type of patellofemoral dysfunction.

Stiffness usually comes on gradually and it is often attributed to 'old age'. It is nothing of the sort; knees only get stiff if there is something wrong with them, and the 'something' is usually osteoarthritis. Characteristically it is worse after periods of inactivity.

Limp is seldom mentioned as a specific complaint, but it often accompanies pain and stiffness.

Locking is an ambiguous term. The joint is not really 'locked' in the sense that it cannot move at all. One minute it moves perfectly well, and the next it gets 'stuck' short of full extension; something (a torn meniscus or a loose body) has got jammed between the articular surfaces. Sudden *unlocking* is even more suggestive; the obstruction has moved and the joint has unjammed.

Swelling, if it appears immediately after an injury, suggests a haemarthrosis due to a torn ligament or a fracture. If it appears only after several hours, it may be due to a torn meniscus. Chronic swelling is usually due to arthritis or synovitis.

Deformity, especially if it is of recent onset, is quickly noticed. It may be unilateral or bilateral; valgus or varus, fixed flexion or hyperextension ('back-knee'). Knock knees and bandy legs are common in children and often correct spontaneously as the child grows up. Progressive deformity in older people suggests arthritis.

Giving way can be due to muscle weakness, but more often it is due to a mechanical disorder, such as a torn ligament or a torn meniscus. Patellar instability is another important cause of giving way.

Loss of function usually appears as diminished walking distance, inability to run, difficulty going up or down stairs, and problems sitting down or rising from a chair.

EXAMINATION

You will have seen something of the gait when the patient came in. For the examination, both lower limbs must be exposed from groins to toes; a mere hitching up of the skirt or rolling back of a trouser leg is not good enough.

The examination is conducted in four stages: with the patient upright (standing and walking); with the patient sitting; with the patient lying on the couch supine; and then lying prone.

With the patient upright

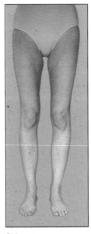
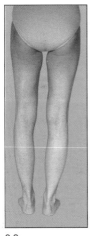

8.1, 8.2 Look at the general shape and posture of the lower limbs. Normally the knees are in very slight valgus, with the patellae pointing directly forwards. Look for scars, or signs of inflammation. Is the knee swollen? Is there muscle wasting above the knee? And don't forget the feet – foot disorders may cause secondary problems in the knee!

8.1   8.2

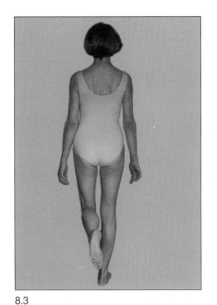

8.3

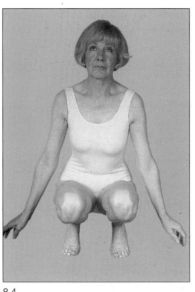

8.4

8.3 Now ask her to walk back and forth several times. Note the rhythm and character of her gait. Pay attention to the knee during the stance phase; does it remain stable or is there a sideways wobble?

8.4 If she can do so without too much pain, ask her to squat; loss of flexion will quickly be revealed.

8.5, 8.6 Deformity, and especially unilateral deformity, is usually more noticeable with the patient standing. The patient in **8.5** has valgus of both knees (and the feet and the big toes); she has rheumatoid arthritis. Bilateral varus (**8.6**) is more common in osteoarthritis.

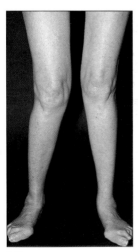

8.5

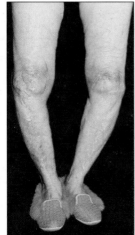

8.6

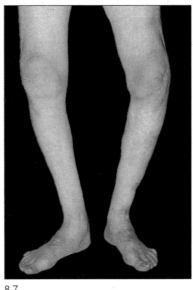

8.7

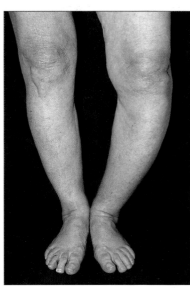

8.8

8.7, 8.8 Both of these patients have varus on the left side. But look more closely. In **8.7** the deformity is in the joint and the knee is grossly unstable; in **8.8** the deformity is in the tibia (due to Paget's disease) and the joint is normal.

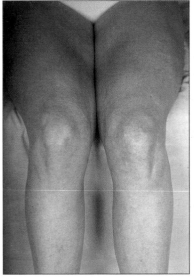

8.9

With the patient sitting

8.9 Ask the patient to sit sideways on the examination couch with her knees over the edge. Look at the shape and position of the patellae. Are the knees symmetrical? Is one patella higher than the other, or is it displaced to one side?

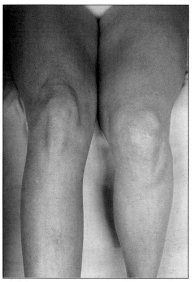 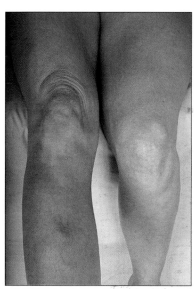

8.10   8.11

8.10, 8.11 Now ask her to straighten each knee in turn, and observe how the patella moves. You can see how, with increasing extension of the knee, the patella normally glides upwards while remaining centred over the femoral condyles. In patellar subluxation, the patella slips or tilts laterally as the knee flexes and then veers back to the midline as the knee extends.

With the patient supine

8.12 Begin by looking at the limb as a whole, comparing it with the opposite side. Concentrate on the skin: is the colour normal, or is there redness (suggesting inflammation)? Look for scars: they are like surgical archaeology – a record of past events. Then compare the knees for signs of swelling or muscle wasting.

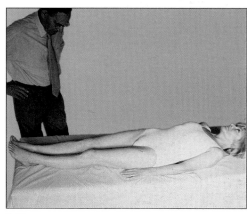

8.12

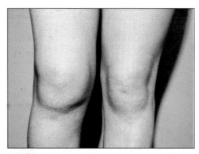

8.13

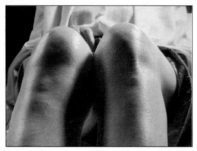

8.14

8.13, 8.14 The patient in **8.13** has diffuse swelling of the right knee; she has rheumatoid synovitis and a large effusion. The patient in **8.14** has a much less obvious effusion. Look carefully at the hollows that normally appear lateral to the patellar ligaments when the knees are partially flexed: on the left side the hollow is there; on the right it is not – there is a small joint effusion.

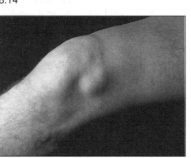

8.15

8.15 Localized swellings are always interesting. The two small lumps are in the joint and they move about. They are cartilaginous loose bodies.

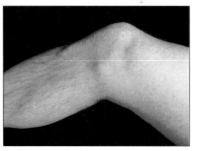

8.16

8.16 This lump is firm, immobile and at the joint line – a cyst of the meniscus.

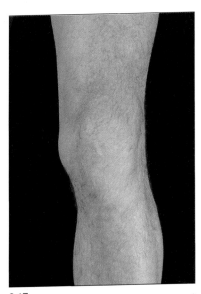

8.17

8.17 In this case the painful swelling is at the proximal end of the medial collateral ligament; it is due to calcification of the ligament.

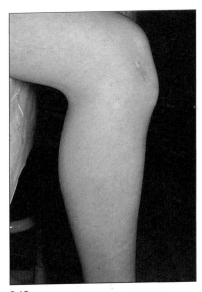

8.18

8.18 Here the tender lump (or 'bump') is way outside the joint, directly over the tibial tubercle. The patient is an athletic young boy with Osgood-Schlatter's disease (osteochondritis of the tibial apophysis).

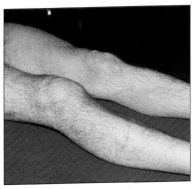

8.19

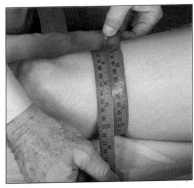

8.20

8.19, 8.20 Wasting of the quadriceps occurs quite rapidly after any internal derangement or disuse of the knee. There is a visible loss of bulk on the right side. Measurement of the girth at the same distance above each knee gives an accurate assessment.

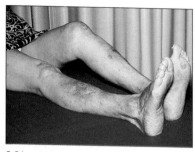

8.21

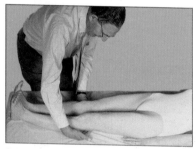

8.22

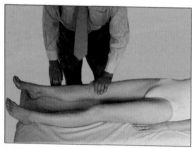

8.23

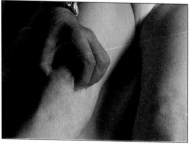

8.24

8.21, 8.22 Look at the position of the knee. Valgus or varus would have been noted before. Is there also a flexion deformity – an inability fully to extend the knee? In **8.21** the deformity is obvious. But in patients with slight abnormalities, the deformity may be difficult to detect. Slide both your hands behind the patient's knees (**8.22**), ask her to press into the couch and then try to slide your hands out. On the normal side your hand will feel trapped, but if there is even a minute flexion deformity it will slide out easily.

8.23 Feeling begins with the skin. Is it warmer than on the normal side? You can compare the two sides by feeling them alternately. You can also slide your hand down the length of the limb; normally it feels steadily cooler as you move distally, and you can easily detect any undue warmth as you reach the knee.

8.24 Feeling the synovial membrane is difficult, but if it is thickened (as in any chronic synovitis) you can detect this by *Solomon's test*: grasp the edges of the patella between your thumb and middle finger and try to lift the patella away from the femur; of course this is impossible, but in the normal knee you have the sense of gripping the patella between your fingers, whereas if the synovium is thickened your fingers will simply slip off the edges of the bone.

8.25, 8.26 Feeling for fluid. The usual test for intra-articular fluid is the *patellar tap*. With your left hand, squeeze out any fluid from the suprapatellar pouch into the main compartment of the joint (**8.25**); if there is a moderate amount of fluid this will lift the patella off the femoral condyles. Maintain the position of your left hand and then, with the fingers of your right hand, push sharply backwards on the patella (**8.26**); with a positive test the patella can be felt striking the femur and bouncing off again (ballottement).

If there is too much fluid, the test will be negative because the patella cannot displace the fluid volume in the joint. But then it should be easy to diagnose the situation by cross fluctuation between the knee joint and the suprapatellar pouch.

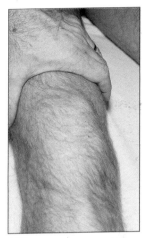

8.25

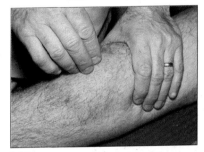

8.26

8.27, 8.28 If there is only a small effusion, the patellar tap also will not work. Here is where you can use the *bulge test*. As in the previous test, first empty the suprapatellar pouch (**8.25**). Then press with your right hand on the medial compartment to displace any fluid towards the lateral side (**8.27**). When you lift your right hand, it may leave a little hollow on the medial side. Now sharply compress the lateral side of the joint (**8.28**); a ripple on the medial side shows that fluid has moved across the joint.

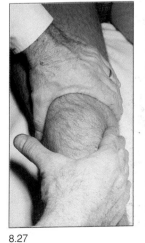

8.27

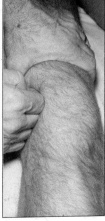

8.28

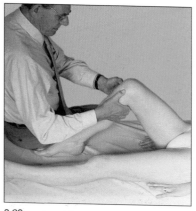

8.29

8.29 Now feel for tenderness. If you can localize the site of tenderness, you are halfway to a diagnosis. Bend both knees to 90° and feel the normal knee first, using your thumbs and fingers. Feel the joint line, the sites of ligament attachment, the patella and the patellar ligament. Repeat this on the affected knee – gently, and watching the patient's face to see if you are hurting her. There is no need to watch your hands, you know where they are!

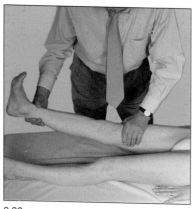

8.30

8.30, 8.31 When examining movement, begin with the knee in full extension (**8.30**); then flex the knee as far as it will go without causing pain (**8.31**). Normally the limit is reached when the calf meets the ham. Any limitation can be recorded either in degrees or by estimating the heel-buttock distance. The normal range is 0–150°.

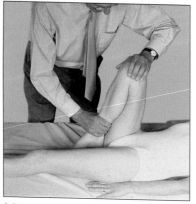

8.31

8.32 Rotation cannot be examined with the knee straight; the knee must be bent. With one hand you feel the knee, with the other you rotate the leg medially and laterally, repeating these movements at various angles of knee flexion. You may feel the click of a torn meniscus and you will see from the patient's face if you are causing pain. If you repeat these movements while exerting a valgus stress on the knee, you are performing *McMurray's test*.

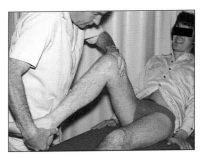

8.32

8.33, 8.34 There are two ways of testing the integrity of the collateral ligaments. **8.33** Grasp the fully extended limb with your left hand immediately above the knee and use your right hand to stress the joint alternately into varus and valgus. The patient shown here has laxity of the medial collateral ligament.
8.34 Alternatively, tuck the patient's ankle under your arm and hold the extended knee with one hand on each side of the joint – your thenar eminences fit nicely into the flare of the upper tibia. Then, with your body, try to angulate the knee into varus and valgus alternately. Significant movement implies abnormal ligamentous laxity.

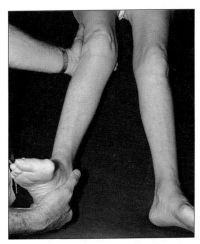

8.33

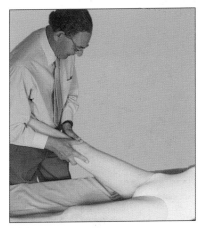

8.34

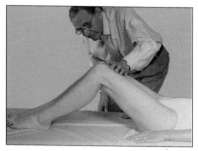

8.35

8.35 The cruciate ligaments are commonly torn at sport, and their integrity can be tested in a number of ways. With the patient's knees flexed 90° and his feet resting on the couch, look at the tibia from the side. If its upper end has dropped back or can be pushed back (the 'sag sign'), the posterior cruciate ligament is torn.

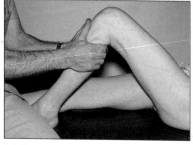

8.36

8.36, 8.37a,b *The 'drawer test'.* With the knee in the same position, stabilize the leg by sitting on the patient's foot. Grasp the top of the patient's leg and try to rock the upper end of the tibia forwards and backwards. The patient may be apprehensive and tighten his hamstrings in order to resist any movement; therefore place your hands high enough to feel these muscles and ensure that they are relaxed. Excessive anterior movement (a positive anterior drawer sign) denotes anterior cruciate ligament laxity; a positive posterior drawer sign denotes posterior cruciate laxity. But if the patient had a positive sag sign, the tibia can be pulled forward to its normal position quite easily; do not be deceived into thinking this is a positive anterior drawer sign – if the tibia comes no further forward than the normal position, it is the posterior cruciate ligament which is stretched or torn. The patient in **8.37a,b** has a positive anterior drawer sign.

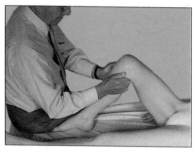

8.37a

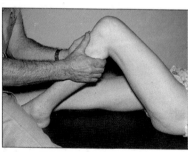

8.37b

8.38 *The Lachman test.* This is more sensitive than the drawer test, but you need big hands. With one hand holding the distal thigh and the other holding the proximal tibia, try to move the tibia backwards and forwards. If movement is greater than in the normal knee, there is cruciate ligament laxity.

Note: There are several special tests for cruciate ligament dysfunction. They are difficult to perform and impossible to illustrate with still photographs. The tests are demonstrated in the videotape recording *Examination of the knee*, by David Dandy (British Orthopaedic Association Videotape Library).

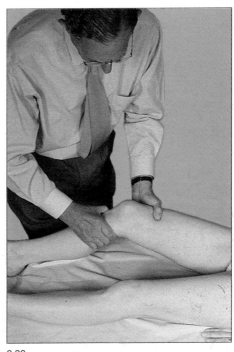

8.38

The patellofemoral joint

8.39 The patellofemoral joint is the source of many knee problems and it merits separate examination. First look to see if the patella is the same shape and in the same position as the patella in the normal knee. It may be smaller than usual, or situated higher than expected (*patella alta*). In the patient shown here, the angle of pull is more valgus on the right side than on the left; this can give rise to mal-tracking of the patella, one of the causes of anterior knee pain.

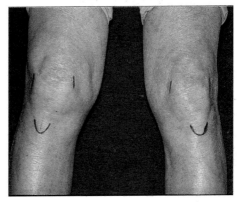

8.39

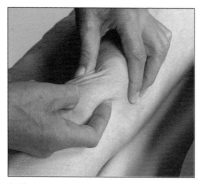

8.40

8.40 Feeling the superficial surface of the patella is seldom rewarding, but the posterior surface is very important. If the quadriceps is relaxed, you can push the patella medially and so feel at least part of the posterior surface, admittedly through skin and synovium. Any roughness or tenderness should be noted. Lateral displacement of the patella is more difficult because of the prominence of the lateral femoral condyle.

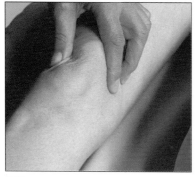

8.41

8.41 A crude test for patellofemoral tenderness is to hold the patella against the femoral condyles and then ask the patient to tighten her thigh muscles; even in normal people this is uncomfortable, but patients with patellofemoral pain will jump with surprise! This is often associated with chondromalacia patellae.

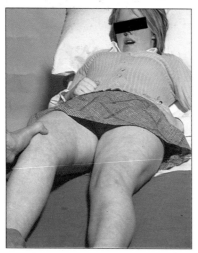

8.42

8.42 *The patellar apprehension test.* Patients with patellar instability (recurrent dislocation or subluxation) may look and feel quite normal between episodes. You can reproduce their symptoms by gently but firmly pushing the patella laterally while slowly bending the knee; the look on this young woman's face betrays her anxiety as she senses that the patella is about to dislocate.

△With the patient prone

8.43 Never forget to examine the back of the joint, so ask the patient to turn over, face downwards, making sure she can breathe comfortably. Look for any scars or swellings.

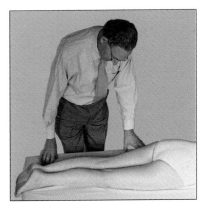

8.43

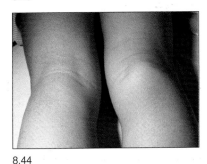

8.44

8.44 This patient has a popliteal 'cyst', due to herniation of the joint capsule; this is sometimes called a *Baker's cyst*.

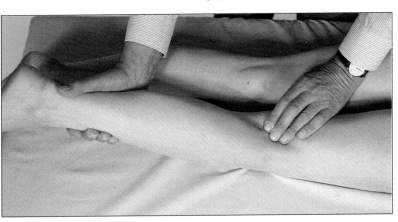

8.45

8.45 Any lump at the back of the knee should be felt carefully, with the muscles relaxed. Bursae and 'cysts' are fluctuant; a popliteal aneurysm pulsates; bone tumours are hard.

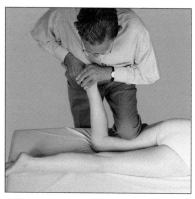

8.46

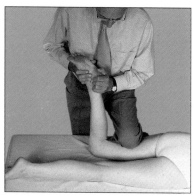

8.47

8.46, 8.47 There are two special tests which are performed with the patient prone, *Apley's 'grinding test'* and *'distraction test'*. With your knee stabilizing the patient's thigh and her knee bent 90°, press on her foot and rotate her leg one way, then the other (**8.46**). Repeat the movements with the knee at different angles of flexion. Pain or clicking suggests meniscal damage.

For the *'distraction test'* (**8.47**), repeat the movements described above, but this time while pulling the patient's leg upwards, so taking pressure off the menisci and tightening the ligaments. If this test is painful, the ligaments are at fault.

9

THE ANKLE
AND FOOT

HISTORY

Pain: 'My feet are killing me'– this prognosis is seldom accurate, but it does indicate the misery which painful feet can cause. The pain may be due to local pathology, but more often it is due to tight shoes or to pressure of the shoe on a bony prominence. So always ask if the patient is comfortable when not wearing shoes and whether the pain follows prolonged standing. With local pathology, often only one foot is affected and the patient can point to the site of the pain. Acute, excruciating pain around the first metatarsophalangeal joint is typical of gout; less often one of the other toes is affected. Pain directly over one of the metatarsal bones, typically arising after a period of strenuous and unaccustomed walking, should suggest a stress fracture. A diffuse ache across the forefoot – *metatarsalgia* – occurs in many different disorders (and sometimes in the normal foot after prolonged standing or walking).

Deformity may be in the ankle, the mid-foot or the toes. Parents often worry about their children being 'flat-footed' or 'pigeon-toed'. Most become normal as the child grows up, but it is difficult to convince the parents of this. Deformity of the foot or toes, worrisome in itself, is also trying because the patient has difficulty fitting shoes.

Swelling may be diffuse and bilateral, or localized. Unilateral swelling nearly always has a 'surgical' cause, bilateral swelling is often 'medical' in origin. Swelling over the medial side of the first metatarsal head (a bunion) is common, especially in older women.

Corns and callosities usually come to light because of tenderness and pressure from shoes.

Numbness and paraesthesia may be felt in all the toes, or only in a circum-scribed area served by a single nerve. Careful enquiry about the distribution of symptoms will yield valuable clues as to whether you are dealing with a local disorder or a more central neurological disorder. 'Dead feet' may be an early symptom of a polyneuritis.

Coldness and colour changes are common complaints in patients with circulatory disorders. A complaint of chronic ulceration should prompt further questions about symptoms of diabetes.

EXAMINATION

At a minimum the lower limbs must be exposed from the thighs down; sometimes it is necessary to have the back exposed as well. The patient needs to be observed facing you, with his back to you, and on tip-toes in both positions. Then he should be watched walking away from you, back towards you, and again on tip-toes in both cases. Don't forget to look at the shoes; providing they are not brand new, the pattern of wear is often informative.

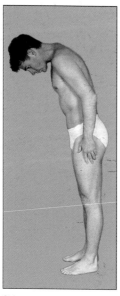

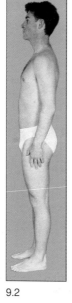

9.1, 9.2 This man knows you are looking at his feet, so he does likewise; if you are bending down to look closely, you may not realize that his feet are not properly balanced. It is best therefore to tell him to look straight in front of him and you should glance up to make sure he does so. Note his posture and the general appearance of his knees and calves. Now look for any scars, abnormalities of colour, corns (which are hard buttons of skin usually on the dorsum of the toe joints) and any undue prominences, such as bunions or an 'overbone', which is an exostosis on the dorsum of the mid-foot. If the patient can point to a definite spot which is painful, that is always helpful.

9.1   9.2

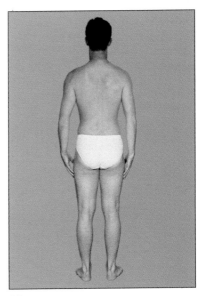

9.3 Look carefully at the position of the ankles and feet with the patient standing. Normally the Achilles tendons and heels are in line with the legs, or perhaps turned slightly outwards. The feet are balanced in the neutral position and the medial (longitudinal) arches are visible but not excessively high.

9.3

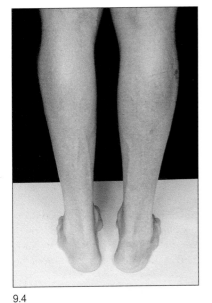

9.4

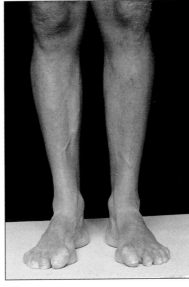

9.5

9.4, 9.5 In this patient the heels are turned inwards (varus) and the longitudinal arches are higher than normal (cavus). Note how this often goes with clawing of the toes and thinning of the calf muscles.

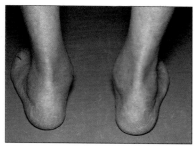

9.6

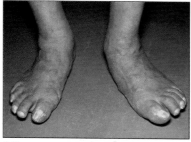

9.7

9.6, 9.7 This is the opposite deformity – flat feet (pes planus). In severe cases the medial arches have disappeared and the heels are everted (plano-valgus). The patient in **9.7** has rheumatoid arthritis.

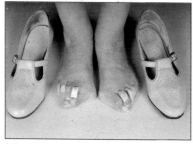

9.8

9.8 Deformities are often confined to the forefoot. The commonest are hallux valgus and claw toes; this woman has both, and her shoes are also mis-shapen.

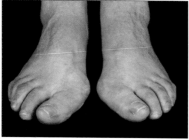

9.9

9.9 This patient with severe hallux valgus has all the classical features of the condition: flattening of the forefeet, lateral deviation and rotation of the big toes, medial angulation of the first metatarsals and prominent, tender bunions.

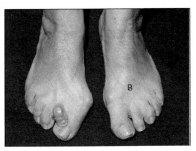

9.10

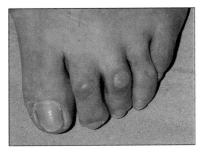

9.11

9.10 In some cases the big toe comes to lie beneath the second toe, causing dorsal subluxation of the second metatarsophalangeal joint and a hammer toe deformity of the second digit.

9.11 In this patient with claw toes there are flexion deformities of both the proximal interphalangeal and the distal interphalangeal joints. She has developed painful corns on the tops of the two middle toes.

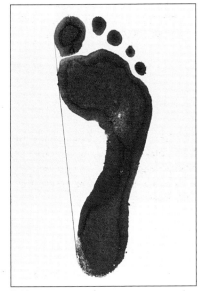

9.12

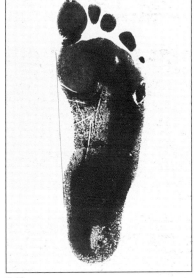

9.13

9.12, 9.13 If, while standing and walking, the patient's feet have picked up some dust from the floor, you have a ready-made footprint. Here we have produced some prints by using an ink-pad. Normally there is a blank area, or hollow, corresponding to the medial arch (**9.12**). If there is no medial hollow in the print, the patient is flat-footed (**9.13**).

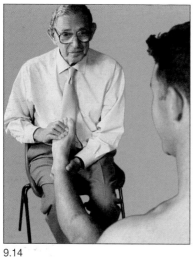

9.14

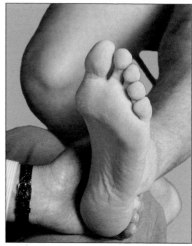

9.15

9.14, 9.15 The examination is continued with the examiner and patient seated. Again you should look for scars, abnormalities of colour, ulceration and corns or callosities. And don't forget the toenails.

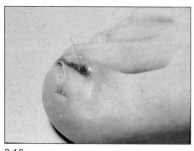

9.16

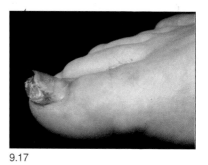

9.17

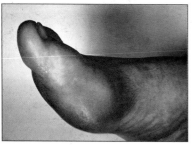

9.18

9.16–9.18 Three painful big-toes: an infected, ingrown toenail (**9.16**); a hard subungual exostosis, which has lifted the nail (**9.17**); and the notorious picture of gout, a painful, inflamed metatarsophalangeal joint (**9.18**).

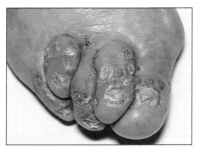

9.19

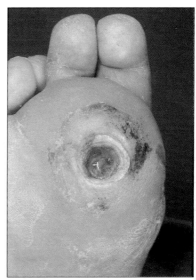

9.20

9.19, 9.20 Skin lesions may be diagnostic: **9.19** shows the features of keratoderma blenorrhagica, a complication of Reiter's disease; **9.20** shows a typical pressure ulcer in a patient with diabetic neuropathy.

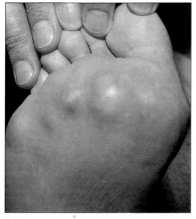

9.21

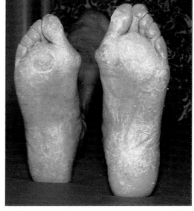

9.22

9.21, 9.22 Look carefully at the soles. Here is where you will see painful bursae and callosities under prominent metatarsal heads. The toes are clawed and the metatarsophalangeal joints are subluxated. The deformities are at first mobile; downward pressure on the metatarsal heads has caused flattening of the transverse metatarsal arch, splaying of the forefoot, and plantar depression of the metatarsal heads. With time these changes become fixed.

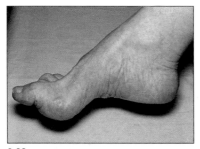

9.23

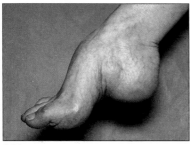

9.24

9.23, 9.24 Check again on the shape and position of each foot. The patient in **9.23** has a cavus deformity; with the foot in repose, the toes are clawed, but they are still passively correctible. A tendon re-balancing procedure might be appropriate. The foot in **9.24** looks similar, but here the high arch is due to severe plantar deviation of the forefoot – a so-called plantaris deformity. The position is fixed and, if correction is needed, this will require major reconstructive surgery.

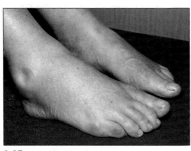

9.25

9.25 Feel for joint swelling, bony lumps and tenderness, remembering to keep looking at the patient's face so that you can detect any sign of pain. This patient has swelling (with pitting) over the peroneal tendon sheath, due to peroneal tenosynovitis.

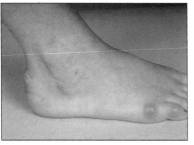

9.26

9.26 This patient has painful 'heel-bumps', due partly to prominence of the calcaneal buttress and partly to a calcaneal bursitis; she also has a tender bump over the fifth meta-tarsophalangeal joint – a so-called bunionette (the counterpart of a medial bunion).

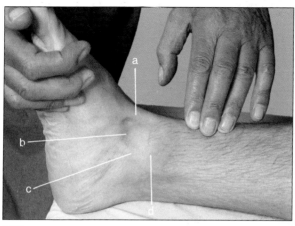

9.27

9.27 Before feeling, it is important to recall the surface anatomy. Knowing precisely which structure is tender goes a long way to revealing the diagnosis. Start with the ankle. By asking the patient to tense his muscles, we can easily identify a number of landmarks: (a) the tendon of tibialis anterior; (b) the depression marking the ankle joint; and (c) the tendon of tibialis posterior running behind the medial malleolus. Just below and slightly anterior to the medial malleolus lies (d) the medial collateral ligament.

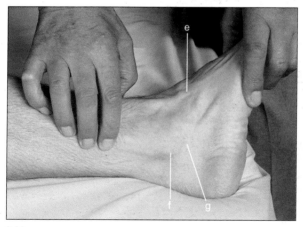

9.28

9.28 On the lateral aspect we can pick out (e) the extensor tendons of the toes and (f) the peroneal tendons curving behind the lateral malleolus. Below the tip of the lateral malleolus lies (g) the lateral collateral ligament.

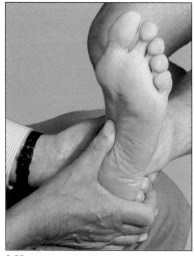

9.29

9.29 Deep pain and tenderness under the medial arch, or a little further back at the edge of the calcaneum, is typical of plantar fasciitis. This is a type of enthesopathy; it is sometimes associated with gout or Reiter's disease, but in most cases no specific cause is found.

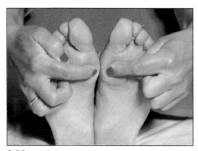

9.30

9.30 This woman is pointing to the spots where, for many years, she had pain on standing. Tenderness was sharply localized to the sesamoid bones, suggesting chondromalacia of the sesamoid-metatarsal joints (sometimes called sesamoiditis).

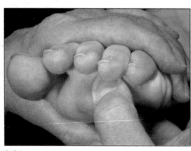

9.31   9.32

9.31, 9.32 The usual site of tenderness in Morton's metatarsalgia. Typically the pain and tenderness are associated with numbness of the adjacent sides of the third and fourth toes. The condition is due to entrapment and thickening of the digital nerve between these two digitis.

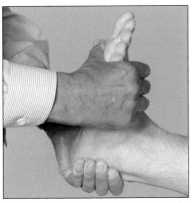
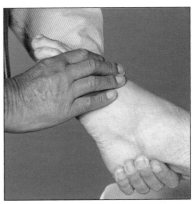

9.33

9.34

9.33, 9.34 Begin with the ankle joint. Grasp the heel with your left hand and the foot with your right. For dorsiflexion, pull down with your left hand and push up with your right. For plantarflexion, pull the foot down with your right hand while retaining your grip on the heel with your left hand. These movements should be examined with the knee slightly flexed so that ankle movement is not impeded by a tight tendo Achillis.

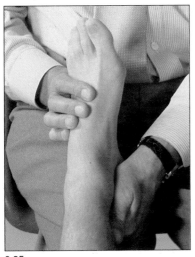
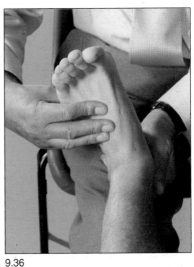

9.35

9.36

9.35, 9.36 Still retaining your grip on the heel and foot, turn the entire foot inwards (inversion) and then outwards (eversion). Inversion normally has a greater range than eversion. Forefoot rotation combined with inversion is called supination; combined with eversion it is called pronation.

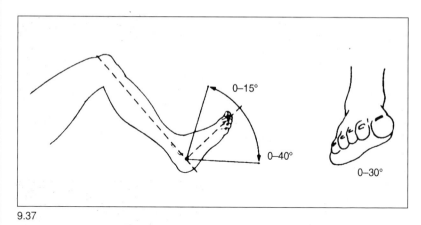

9.37

9.37 The normal ranges of ankle and subtalar movement.

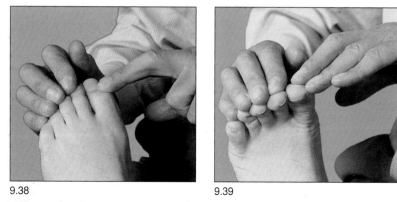

9.38   9.39

9.38, 9.39 Movements of the toes should be tested separately. For brevity, flexion and extension are examined here as mass movements.

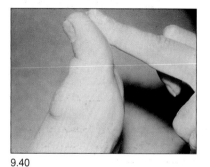

9.40

9.40 Doctors love Latin names! A very stiff big-toe metatarsophalangeal joint is called (unsurprisingly) *hallux rigidus*. It is usually due to osteoarthritis. Extension (dorsiflexion) is impossible and the patient may compensate for this by hyper-extending the interphalangeal joint.

9.41 The integrity of the large tendons around the ankle should be assessed by asking the patient to move the ankle and foot actively against resistance in the direction served by each tendon in turn. Here we demonstrate how to examine the tendon of tibialis posterior, which is the one that ruptures most frequently. Ask the patient to 'point your toes, then turn your foot inwards while I push against the foot'. The tibialis posterior is the main invertor in plantarflexion; you can see the tendon standing out clearly below the medial malleolus.

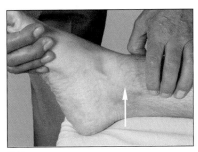
9.41

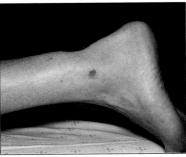

9.42 The calf and ankle may need to be examined with the patient lying prone. In this patient, who had 'weakness' of the ankle, there is an obvious dent in the tendo Achillis. He has an old rupture of the tendon.

9.42

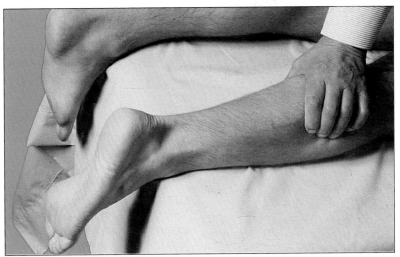

9.43

9.43 Achilles tendon rupture is not always so easily detected. *Simmonds' test* is diagnostic. Normally, when the calf is squeezed the foot automatically plantarflexes; if the tendon is ruptured, this fails to occur.

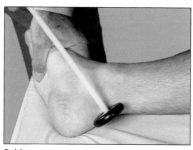
9.44

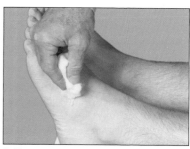
9.45

9.44, 9.45 If the symptoms are suggestive, a complete neurological examination should be performed. Abnormal sensibility, trophic changes, unexplained ulceration and deformities such as claw-toes or drop-foot are characteristic features in various neuropathies.

INDEX